BTEC National Health and Social Care

Book 2

Specialist units

Mary Crittenden
Elizabeth Rasheed

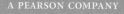
A PEARSON COMPANY

Contents

1121969

How to use this book

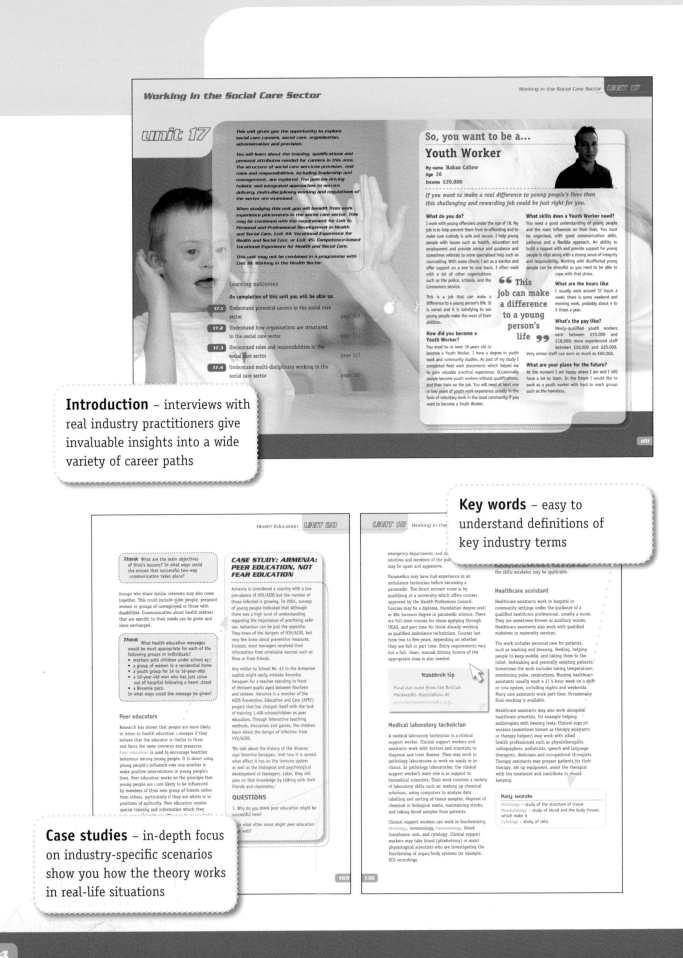

Introduction – interviews with real industry practitioners give invaluable insights into a wide variety of career paths

Key words – easy to understand definitions of key industry terms

Case studies – in-depth focus on industry-specific scenarios show you how the theory works in real-life situations

Grading criteria – learning outcomes and grading criteria are located at the beginning of every unit, so you know right from the start what you need to do to achieve a pass, merit or distinction

UNIT 12 Public Health

Grading criteria

The table shows what you need to do to gain a pass, merit or distinction in this part of the qualification. Make sure you refer back to it when you are completing work so you can judge whether you are meeting the criteria and what you need to do to fill in gaps in your knowledge or experience.

In this unit there are four evidence activities that give you an opportunity to demonstrate your achievement of the grading criteria

page 75	P1
page 83	P2
page 91	P3, P4, M1 and D1
page 99	P5, P6, M2, M3 and D2

To achieve a pass grade the evidence must show that the learner is able to...	To achieve a merit grade the evidence must show that, in addition to the pass criteria, the learner is able to...	To achieve a distinction grade the evidence must show that, in addition to the pass and merit criteria, the learner is able to...
P1 Describe key aspects of public health in the UK		
P2 Describe the origins of public health in the UK		
P3 Identify current patterns of ill health and inequality in the UK	M1 Explain probable causes of the current patterns of ill health and inequality in the UK	D1 Evaluate the role of factors that contribute to the current patterns of ill health and inequality in the UK
P4 Describe six factors that potentially affect health status in the UK		
P5 Describe methods of promoting and protecting public health	M2 Explain methods of promoting and protecting public health	
P6 Identify appropriate methods of prevention/control for a named communicable disease and a named non-communicable disease.	M3 Explain appropriate methods of prevention/control for a named communicable disease and a named non-communicable disease.	D2 Evaluate the effectiveness of methods of promoting and protecting public health for the two named diseases.

Evidence activities – short activities are spread throughout the unit giving you the opportunity to practice your achievement of the grading criteria in small steps

Think – questions help you reflect on your learning and to think about how it could be applied to real-life working practice

UNIT 20 Health Education

Research tip

You can find out more from Emil Sahakyan, Communication Officer, UNICEF Armenia: www.unicef.org/armenia/realives_2856.html

Research tip

Log on to NHS Direct to get health information at www.nhsdirect.nhs.uk

EVIDENCE ACTIVITY

P1 – M1

P1 Explain three different approaches to health education.

M1 Compare three different approaches to health education.

Choose three health education campaigns that use different approaches. Describe and compare each of the campaigns, including the subject matter and the approach that is used. Were they appropriate for the campaign and why was one approach chosen above another?

Theatre and drama

Another way of approaching health education is through the use of theatre and drama. Messages can be conveyed directly or indirectly as part of a story line. The development of skills and confidence can often be enhanced through the use of drama. Sensitive subjects may be expressed through drama; for example, theatre groups have spread health messages among Mozambique's flood victims.

Finally as computers and videos become more interactive they can be used as a method of two-way communication. Interactive packages offer health assessments. Video can facilitate live discussions and may be used to provide information.

Figure 20.4 Children in Mozambique, captivated by a play, learn important skills from community activists.

Research tips – direct you to useful websites and key organisations to help you take your study further

Health Education UNIT 20

20.2 Understand models of behaviour change

MODELS

The ultimate aim of any health education is to change people's behaviour so that they lead healthier lives. However, it is not always straightforward to get individuals to adopt healthy behaviours and the process of making any change can be complex. The various stages through which individuals change are described in a number of different models.

Health belief model

The health belief model is one of the best known. It suggests that:

- an individual must believe that they are susceptible to a certain disease
- the disease is serious
- the proposed preventative action will be beneficial
- the benefits will outweigh any costs or disadvantages
- they are competent to carry out the behaviour
- the likelihood of action will be enhanced if the individual has a positive view of health
- cues or triggers to action are provided.

Example

Simon is in his first year at university. He is shocked to hear that one of his fellow students has developed meningitis and is very ill. The university has distributed a number of leaflets giving information about the disease. Simon realises that his age group is at particular risk. The medical centre is offering immunisation to all students. However Simon does not like needles.

Think Use the health belief model to see if you can predict whether Simon will attend the medical centre and why.

Theory of reasoned action

Fishbein and Ajzen proposed the theory of reasoned action. They suggested that behaviour can be predicted by knowing what someone intends to do. An intention is formed by a person's attitude to the behaviour and their perception of what other people will think about them if they behave in a certain way (subjective norms). This model recognises that the attitudes of other people can also have an effect on the behaviour of an individual.

Figure 20.5 The health belief model (Source: Glanz, K., Rimer, B.K. & Lewis, F.M. (2002). Health Behavior and Health Education: theory, Research and Practice. San Francisco: Wiley & Sons).

Examples – industry-specific examples show you what the theory looks like in practice

Track your progress

This master grid can be used as a study aid. You can track your progress by ticking the level you achieve. The relevant grading criteria can also be found at the start of each unit.

To achieve a pass grade the evidence must show that the learner is able to...	To achieve a merit grade the evidence must show that, in addition to the pass criteria, the learner is able to...	To achieve a distinction grade the evidence must show that, in addition to the pass and merit criteria, the learner is able to...
Unit 9		
P1 describe the processes of care planning with reference to care planning principles	**M1** explain care planning principles	
P2 identify the importance of multi-disciplinary and inter-agency working on the care planning process	**M2** use examples to explain how multi-disciplinary and inter-agency working can improve the care planning process	**D1** evaluate the role of multi-disciplinary and inter-agency working in social care
P3 use four examples to describe key aspects of legislation, policies and codes of practice that influence social care	**M3** explain the impact of legislation on the concept of care planning	**D2** evaluate the effectiveness of current legislation in promoting care planning and multi-disciplinary/inter-agency working.
P4 describe the values that underpin social care practice		
P5 describe ethical principles in relation to social care	**M4** explain the roles of individuals and organisations in relation to values and ethical practice	
Unit 11		
P1 explain how individual rights can be respected in a supportive relationship	**M1** explain how supportive relationships can enhance the life experiences of individuals receiving health and social care services	**D1** use examples to evaluate the role of supportive relationships in enhancing the life experiences of individuals receiving heath and social care services
P2 describe different forms of abuse that may be experienced by vulnerable adults		
P3 describe different indicators of abuse in vulnerable adults		
P4 describe the potential for abuse in health and social care contexts	**M2** analyse the potential for abuse in four health and social care contexts	
P5 describe strategies and working practices used to minimise abuse		
P6 identify the legislation, policies and procedures that protect adults receiving health and social care services.	**M3** explain how legislation, policies and procedures contribute to the protection of vulnerable adults	**D2** analyse the role of multi-agency working in minimising the risks of abuse in health and social care contexts.

To achieve a pass grade the evidence must show that the learner is able to...	To achieve a merit grade the evidence must show that, in addition to the pass criteria, the learner is able to...	To achieve a distinction grade the evidence must show that, in addition to the pass and merit criteria, the learner is able to...
Unit 12		
P1 describe key aspects of public health in the UK		
P2 describe the origins of public health in the UK		
P3 identify current patterns of ill health and inequality in the UK	**M1** explain probable causes of the current patterns of ill health and inequality in the UK	**D1** evaluate the role of factors that contribute to the current patterns of ill health and inequality in the UK
P4 describe six factors that potentially affect health status in the UK		
P5 describe methods of promoting and protecting public health	**M2** explain methods of promoting and protecting public health	
P6 identify appropriate methods of prevention/control for a named communicable disease and a named non-communicable disease.	**M3** explain appropriate methods of prevention/control for a named communicable disease and a named non-communicable disease	**D2** evaluate the effectiveness of methods of promoting and protecting public health for two named diseases.
Unit 17		
P1 describe the requirements for two careers in the social care sector	**M1** explain how the requirements of social care workers can contribute to providing a positive experience for service users	**D1** evaluate the requirements of social care workers in terms of providing a competent workforce in social care services
P2 describe the overall structure of social care provision in home country		
P3 describe the roles and responsibilities of three overarching organisations in social care	**M2** explain the roles of three organisations in improving social care service provision	
P4 describe three examples of legislation, policies, standards or codes of practice that influence social care service provision	**M3** explain the role of legislation, policies, standards or codes of practice in improving social care provision	
P5 explain the role of workforce development in social care sector		
P6 describe two examples of multi-disciplinary working in social care	**M4** explain how multi-disciplinary working can improve social care service provision	**D2** use examples to evaluate the effectiveness of multi-disciplinary working for service users

To achieve a pass grade the evidence must show that the learner is able to...	To achieve a merit grade the evidence must show that, in addition to the pass criteria, the learner is able to...	To achieve a distinction grade the evidence must show that, in addition to the pass and merit criteria, the learner is able to...
Unit 18		
P1 describe the requirements for two careers in the health sector	**M1** explain how requirements of health care workers can contribute to providing a positive experience for patients	**D1** evaluate the requirements of health care workers in terms of providing a competent workforce for the health sector
P2 describe the overall structure of health services provision in home country		
P3 describe the roles and responsibilities of three overarching organisations in the health sector	**M2** explain the roles of the three organisations in improving health services provision	
P4 describe three examples of legislation, policies, standards or codes of practice that influence provision of health services	**M3** explain the role of legislation, policies, standards or codes of practice in improving provision of health services	
P5 explain the role of workforce development in the health sector		
P6 describe two examples of multi-disciplinary working in the health sector	**M4** explain how multi-disciplinary working can improve the provision of health services	**D2** use examples to evaluate the effectiveness of multi-disciplinary working for patients
Unit 20		
P1 explain three different approaches to health education	**M1** compare three different approaches to health education	
P2 describe two different models of behaviour change and the importance of the social and economic context		
P3 describe the design and implementation of own small scale health education campaign	**M2** explain the approaches and methods used in own health education campaign, relating them to models of behaviour change	**D1** evaluate the approaches and methods used in own health education campaign relating them to models of behaviour change
P4 explain how own health education campaign met the aims and objectives and explain the ethical issues involved	**M3** analyse how own health education campaign met aims and objectives and addressed any ethical issues	
P5 explain how own small scale health education campaign links to local/national/international targets and strategies for health.	**M4** analyse the role of own small scale health education campaign in terms of local/national/international targets and strategies for health	**D1** evaluate own health education campaign.

Research Skills

Before you start your research project you need to know where to find information and the guidelines you must follow.

Types of information

Primary Sources

Information you have gathered yourself, through surveys, interviews, photos or observation. Ensure that you ask the appropriate questions and people. You must get permission before including someone's photo or interview in your work.

Secondary Sources

Information produced by somebody else, including information from the internet, books, magazines, databases and television. You need to be sure that your secondary source is reliable if you are going to use the information.

Information Sources

The Internet

The internet is a useful research tool, but, not all the information you find will be. When using the internet ask yourself if you can trust the information you find.

> Acknowledge your source! When quoting from the internet always include author name (if known)/document title/URL web address/date site was accessed.

Books, Magazines and Newspapers

Information in newspapers and magazines is up to date and usually researched thoroughly. Books have a longer shelf life than newspapers so make sure you use the most recent edition.

> Acknowledge your source! When quoting from books, magazines, journal or papers, always include author name/ title of publication/publisher/year of publication.

Broadcast Media

Television and radio broadcast current news stories and the information should be accurate. Be aware that some programmes offer personal opinions as well as facts.

Plagiarism

Plagiarism is including in your own work extracts or ideas from another source without acknowledging its origins. If you use any material from other sources you must acknowledge it. This includes the work of fellow students.

Storing Information

Keep a record of all the information you gather. Record details of book titles, author names, page references, web addresses (URLs) and contact details of interviewees. Accurate, accessible records will help you acknowledge sources and find information quickly.

Internet Dos and Don'ts

Do ✔

- check information against other sources
- keep a record of where you found information and acknowledge the source
- be aware that not all sites are genuine or trustworthy

Don't ∅

- assume all the information on the internet is accurate and up to date
- copy material from websites without checking whether permission from the copyright holder is required
- give personal information to people you meet on the internet

Values and Planning in Social Care

unit 9

In this unit you will learn about care planning in social care. Planning is needed to make sure that care happens as it should. Good planning helps to make sure that care is effective – that it does what it is supposed to do. Care planning must be efficient, delivering as much care as possible without wasting resources. Those who plan care must follow guidelines set out in laws, policies and codes of practice. Laws such as the Human Rights Act, the Disability Discrimination Act, Health and Safety at Work and the Data Protection Act, are just some of the issues to be considered when planning care.

Values and ethical principles also influence the planning process and span political, social and cultural differences. Some politicians think people should pay for their own care. Others think the state should provide and the money should come from taxpayers. Some people have better health because of their lifestyle, income and the choices they make. Culturally, some people will not want to visit the doctor while others will visit every time they have a cold. In care, difficult decisions have to be made. Resources are limited and not every need can be met. Care workers must balance the needs of individuals with the resources that are available while at the same time upholding and respecting the rights of people. This unit will introduce you to some of the issues at the centre of care today.

Learning outcomes

On completion of this unit you will be able to:

So, you want to be a...

Care Manager

My name Priya Mattu
Age 35
Income £26,000

If you are good at managing budgets and people and want to help people lead an independent life, this could be the job for you...

What does a Care manager do?

I work in a care home for elderly people; I assess the needs of clients and commission the services they need. I manage individual case loads and work in partnership with social services and health care organisations. A good Care Manager can really make a difference to people's lives and help them maintain independence and lead more fulfilling lives. I am fully accountable for my own practice and I am responsible for staff training too.

How did you get into the job?

Many care managers have a nursing or social work qualification before they become care managers but I become a care manager through the NVQ route. I had a lot of practical experience in the care sector and I took a Level 4 Registered Manager's award, before landing this job.

What skills do you need?

You must be good at a communicating with and managing different people. Computer skills are very important because accurate record keeping is essential and you need to be able to understand and manage budgets. You should be able to cope well with stress and should like working with older people. All care workers need to have a Criminal Records Bureau check and be cleared to work with vulnerable adults under POVA regulations.

What are the hours like?

I sometimes have to work long hours if workers are off sick and there is not enough replacement cover. I also have to work some weekends and bank holidays, and occasionally work at night.

> **" A good Care Manager can really make a difference to people's lives "**

What is the pay like?

The pay is not particularly high and varies depending on where you work; you will earn more in the south east of England for example. An experienced Care manager can earn around £30,000 but it's not a job you go into just for the money.

What does the future hold?

I may decide to move to managing a larger unit, but at the moment I am happy where I am. A move into management in the private sector is also an option.

Grading criteria

The table below shows what you need to do to gain a pass, merit or distinction in this part of the qualification. Make sure you refer back to it when you are completing work so you can judge whether you are meeting the criteria and what you need to do to fill in gaps in your knowledge or experience.

In this unit there are four evidence activities that give you an opportunity to demonstrate your achievement of the grading criteria:

page 25   P1, P2, M1, M2 and D1

page 31   P3

page 33   M3 and D2

page 39   P4, P5 and M4

To achieve a pass grade the evidence must show that the learner is able to...	To achieve a merit grade the evidence must show that, in addition to the pass criteria, the learner is able to...	To achieve a distinction grade the evidence must show that, in addition to the pass and merit criteria, the learner is able to...
P1 Describe the processes of care planning with reference to care planning principles	**M1** Explain care planning principles	
P2 Identify the importance of multi-disciplinary and inter-agency working on the care planning process	**M2** Use examples to explain how multi-disciplinary and inter-agency working can improve the care planning process	**D1** Evaluate the role of multi-disciplinary and inter-agency working in social care
P3 Use four examples to describe key aspects of legislation, policies and codes of practice that influence social care	**M3** Explain the impact of legislation on the concept of care planning	**D2** Evaluate the effectiveness of current legislation in promoting care planning and multi-disciplinary/inter-agency working
P4 Describe the values that underpin social care practice		
P5 Describe ethical principles in relation to social care	**M4** Explain the roles of individuals and organisations in relation to values and ethical practice	

9.1 *Care planning principles and processes*

CASE STUDY: LORRAINE

Lorraine is 17 years old and is currently homeless. Until the age of 13 she lived with her mother; her father left the family home when Lorraine was younger and she no longer has any contact with him. At the age of 13 Lorraine spent a year in care after she and her mother struggled to live together. After one year Lorraine returned to her mother's but the relationship was still strained and after several arguments Lorraine left home again. Lorraine spent a few weeks sleeping at friends' houses but this was not a long term solution and she had to keep moving on. Eventually when Lorraine had run out of places to stay she started sleeping rough. Lorraine eventually contacted her social worker and moved to a supported housing scheme. Lorraine struggled to get on with the other young people there and after several incidents, she was evicted and went back on the streets.

Lorraine is not her real name, but the problems in this case study are real. As we work through this unit, think how you could apply the ideas to Lorraine's case.

PRINCIPLES

The care planning principles outlined below are important to make sure that the care offered to clients and patients is consistent and is fit for purpose. If there were no guiding principles the quality and quantity of care offered would vary with different care professionals. Service users would not be treated fairly.

Key words

service user, client and patient – all terms for a person who uses the service. 'Patient' is used in health care. 'Service user' and 'client' are often used in social care.

Empowerment of service user

One of the first principles of care planning is that the service user should be empowered (given power) by having a chance to say what they want and how they feel. It is important that care is not simply 'done' to someone, but rather that they are involved in planning their own care.

Needs

From the case study we can see that Lorraine obviously needs somewhere to live but decisions must not be made for her. She must be included in the planning.

Choice

Lorraine should be given a choice of where she lives. Perhaps she is studying at school or college. She may want somewhere close to where she studies, or close to friends. It is important that whenever possible service users are given choice. If Lorraine is given a choice of where to live, she may settle in more quickly and develop a stable routine which enables her to succeed in her new life.

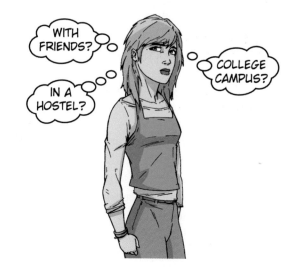

Figure 9.1 Lorraine has many choices to make

Confidentiality

Another principle of care planning is confidentiality. Lorraine's situation is a matter for her and her care team – not for everyone in her class. Those involved with Lorraine's care must not discuss her situation with those who do not have right to the information, so friends who ask about her will not be given details of where she lives.

Rights

Lorraine has the right to tell her friends where she is, but care workers cannot do so. Friends who want to know why she left home will have to ask her themselves. The care team is not allowed to disclose that information.

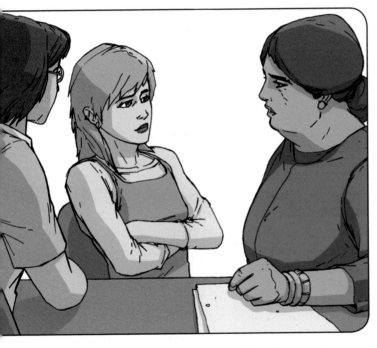

Figure 9.2 Service users such as Lorraine have the right to have their views heard.

Values

The values underpinning care are respect for the client as an individual with individual needs. The service must promote anti-discriminatory practice, offering a confidential service which promotes and supports individual rights. The service must acknowledge individual personal beliefs and identities, and offer this service through effective communication.

Cycle of assessment/planning

Lorraine's social worker would talk to Lorraine and assess her needs. A care plan would be written to meet her needs for shelter and a safe place to stay. The care plan would be reviewed with Lorraine and the care team. Her views would be heard. She may not like the accommodation she has, or she may not have enough money to get to college. The further needs would be assessed and the care plan updated by Lorraine's social worker. The cycle of assessment, planning and review would continue until Lorraine left care.

Key words

care plan – a plan made to meet the needs of an individual. A care plan starts by assessing what a person needs, and then the plan says how the needs will be met. The plan is monitored regularly and evaluated to check that needs are being met. As needs change, the care plan is amended. The care plan should be made by a professional care worker, such as a nurse or social worker, working with the service user. An advocate may represent the views of the service user if the service user wishes.

Potential use of advocates

If they are unable to speak for themselves, service users may have an advocate, someone who speaks on their behalf. Lorraine might have a learning mentor or a Connexions advisor who would represent her views.

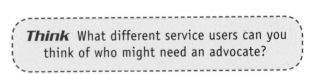

Think What different service users can you think of who might need an advocate?

Service user at the centre of the process

It is a principle of care planning that the service user is at the centre of the process, involved at each stage of the process, fully involved with and aware of what decisions are made and why they are made.

APPROACHES TO CARE PLANNING

Needs-led

A needs-led approach to care planning looks first at the needs of the client. Lorraine needs a safe place to stay, somewhere to call home, so her needs lead the planning process. When Lorraine was homeless at 13, her need for safety was the most important. There was no conflict between what she wanted and what the service could offer. Her assessment was needs-led, but the needs could be met. At 17, again needing a place to stay, she was given a place in a supported housing scheme. Unfortunately she could not get on with the other people living there, and once more found herself homeless.

Service-led

Service-led approaches occur when people want more than a service can offer, for example, an older person may want a home-help to clean their house. In this case, the service is not available from social services. Clients must pay if they want a cleaner. A social worker may be able to offer a carer to help the older person with personal hygiene. This is an example of service-led provision. The service offered may not meet the desires of the client.

Example

In Lorraine's case, she wanted a place to stay but also wanted to please herself and do what she wanted. When you live with other people you have to compromise and think of others. Lorraine quarrelled with the people she shared a house with. We do not know why. She may have wanted to play her music loudly when others were trying to sleep, or she may have been trying to study and the others may have made this impossible. Whatever the reasons, Lorraine again became homeless, but this time we see service-led provision. The service can offer a house but not compatible housemates. Lorraine has been offered shared accommodation but is not happy. She has been evicted, thrown out because of fighting.

Her social worker suggested applying to the council as homeless because, at 17, she should be classed as a priority need. She was provided with temporary accommodation while the housing team carried out an assessment. However, the council has decided that, by causing problems, Lorraine has made herself intentionally homeless. She has been given four weeks to quit her accommodation.

POTENTIAL CONFLICTS

Conflicts arise when there are not enough resources or when people do not respect the rights of others.

Resources

Resources include physical resources such as hostels and also human resources such as carers. Time and money are both resources in short supply.

The council has a few hostels and shared houses for young people but resources are limited.

Rights and responsibilities of service user

Service users such as Lorraine have rights, so at 17 years old, she has the right to a roof over her head, but rights have to be balanced with responsibilities. Lorraine has a responsibility to try to get on with her housemates. If she finds she cannot get on with them, she should talk to her social worker and explain the problem, not quarrel or fight. Lorraine has to take responsibility for her actions and for making herself homeless.

Rights and responsibilities of family/ others

The social worker in this case has a responsibility to represent Lorraine's views, but also a right to expect Lorraine to behave in an acceptable way. Some might think that Lorraine's mother had a responsibility to teach Lorraine how to get along with others.

> ***Think*** Whose responsibility is it to teach children how to behave?
> Should Lorraine's mother have done this?
> Should she offer her a home now?
> Do you think Lorraine's father should have had some share in her upbringing? Should he help her find somewhere to live?

Risk

Lorraine has been evicted to protect the rights of others in the house. She has shown herself to be a risk to others. Social workers and carers have a duty of care to all service users. They cannot allow Lorraine to threaten others.

SKILLS REQUIRED

Care workers need many skills to help service users. These can include:

- excellent communication skills

- being able to build a good relationship

- counselling skills

- effectively planning and implementing care plans

- patience and tolerance.

> ***Think*** What skills do you think are most important in care work?

There are many more skills too. Let's look at each of these and see why they may be needed.

If you have already completed Unit 1, you may already know about effective communication. Much of our communication is non-verbal – that is, we do not have to say it. Lorraine will look at her social worker and decide very quickly whether she will

trust her. This decision will be based on factors such as whether the social worker seems friendly or 'stand-offish' or what her body language is saying. Clothes say a lot. If Lorraine's social worker arrives in a smart office suit, looking like a headmistress, Lorraine might think of her last time at school and decide she does not like what she sees. Effective communication involves overcoming any barriers. The social worker must put Lorraine at her ease yet retain professional boundaries.

Key words

body language – messages are sent out by our non-verbal communication, through the way we stand, sit or look at another person; for example, crossing your arms can make you look defensive or closed to ideas

> ***Think*** What builds a good relationship?
> Who do you tell your problems to? Why do you choose that person?
> What is it about them that encourages you to talk to them?

You may have said they are a good listener; they are always there for you. A good social worker will have these skills. But a social worker is not a friend. A social worker has a duty of care to the client and also has a legal duty to the government.

Trust is essential for good care planning. The service user must feel they can be open with their social worker. A social worker should have good listening skills, but a social worker is not a counsellor. It is important that both Lorraine and her social worker do not confuse the role. Lorraine may need a counsellor, and the social worker will list this as part of the care plan, but the social worker is there to assess Lorraine's needs and plan to meet those needs – not to meet just one need. A social worker must keep an overview of the whole care package.

PROCESSES OF CARE PLANNING

A care plan is just what it says – a plan of how people unable to care for themselves will be cared for.

Care planning cycle

Care planning is often described as a cycle, although a spiral is a more accurate description of what happens. Imagine the cycle below supported by a variety of legislation and guidelines.

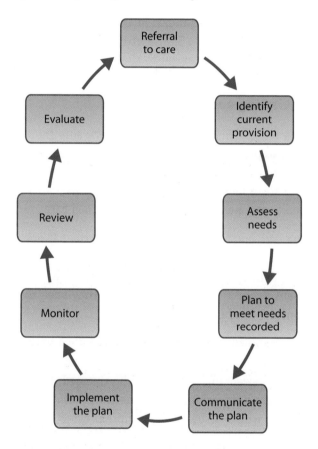

Figure 9.3 The care planning cycle

Referral

Referral is the first stage of the process. People can refer themselves. This is known as self referral. Often they are referred by others. Sometimes a doctor or nurse will refer an older person who is about to be discharged from hospital. Sometimes relatives refer people. Parents caring for grown up children with learning disabilities may make a referral when they feel they can no longer manage to care for their children.

Assessing holistic needs and preferences

This unit is focused on planning in social care, but it is important to remember that care planning also occurs in health care. The client is a whole person and needs cannot be separated. Effective care planning looks at the whole person. This is a holistic approach. Needs and preferences are holistic. An older person who is terminally ill has health needs and social needs that are intertwined. They may need help with washing and dressing but also need pain relief. They may be ill but prefer to die at home rather than in hospital or in a hospice.

In Lorraine's case, her care plan at 13 included arrangements for her:

- placement
- health
- education
- race
- religion and culture
- contact with family and friends.

This is a holistic assessment. Lorraine's physical needs for shelter and safety are identified but so are her social and emotional needs. Contact with friends and family is maintained if it is safe to do so and if she wishes. Her intellectual needs are identified and met by arranging for her education. Lorraine's preferences must be taken into account when planning. By law she has to have an education until she is 16, but she may prefer to move to a college rather than another school.

> **Key words**
> ------------------------------------
> holistic – looking at the whole person and their physical, intellectual, emotional and social needs

Identifying current provision

It is important to identify what is currently provided and how effective that provision is. A person who is terminally ill may have some support from family and friends and they may wish to continue that support with extra help from social services.

Care planning

Care planning is used for anyone who needs care. They may include older people, people with learning disabilities, people with acute and long-term health problems, and people with mental health issues. They may have multiple needs, for an example, an older person with learning disabilities may have a long-term health problem such as asthma. Care planning makes sure the care they get is planned.

Recording

Accurate recording is vital when planning care because the care plan is a legal document which may be used in evidence in a court of law. All written communication records must be factual, not based on hearsay. They should be readable, signed and dated by all parties. Permanent ink should be used and any changes made by crossing through with one line and signing at the side. It must be written in language that the client understands. The care worker must make sure the client's views are accurately represented. The client should sign the care plan.

Communicating

The agencies identified in the care plan should be contacted by the care worker as soon as possible. Confidentiality must be maintained when communicating, so that information passed to another agency is only done so in a secure manner, to a named person. Fax is not acceptable. Anyone may pick up a fax.

Think Why is confidentiality so important?

Implementing

The care plan is implemented, or put into effect, when the carer organises the care. A nurse completing a care plan on a hospital ward may only need to make sure that the immediate care staff are aware of the care needs and carry them out. This may be the needs for hourly drinks, or two hourly turns for an immobile patient. A social worker organising domiciliary care for an older person living alone may need to contact a private care agency and arrange for twice daily visits, as well as the provision of aids such as a grab rail over the bath. The social worker may also organise a visit to a day centre twice a week and may need to set up the transport arrangements.

Monitoring

The care plan must be monitored to make sure that the care happens and to sort out any problems. For example, an older person living alone may be reluctant to have strangers in the house and may not let the carers in. Transport may fail to arrive so the client does not get to the day centre.

Reviewing and evaluating

Care plans should be reviewed to make sure the care originally planned is still needed. Care needs change. Sometimes people have increased needs for care. Sometimes they move away to live with family and no longer require the planned care.

The care must be evaluated. Is it effective? If not, why not? Are two visits a day too much because the client can now mobilise better? Or is the client's condition getting worse and they need to consider residential care?

The care plan is monitored by the social worker to make sure that everything happens as planned. It is reviewed and may have to be changed if plans are not working. This is done at statutory review, which is the legally required review process outlined below.

- The first review is within four weeks of the child being looked after

- The second review will be within three months of the first

- After that they will be on a six monthly basis until the child is no longer looked after.

Key words

statutory – required by law as imposed, for example, by an Act of Parliament

The social worker must record the needs and how they are to be met on the care plan. Each review must be recorded on the plan.

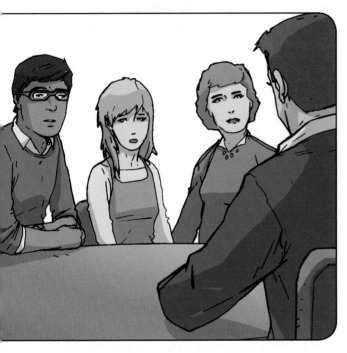

Figure 9.4 The care plan must be monitored and reviewed regularly

Complying with legislation/guidelines

Care planning is used for people who need care. Children and young people looked after by social services are subject to a Care Order, when they are accommodated by the local authority under section 20 of the 1989 Children Act where no one is available to provide care and accommodation and the child or the parent request it.

Social workers must comply with a lot of legislation and guidelines. These include:

- Care Standards Act 2000
- Children Act 2004
- equal opportunities legislation and policies
- General Social Care Council/Care Council for Wales/Northern Ireland Social Care council codes of practice,
- national service frameworks.

Multi-disciplinary working/inter-agency working

A multi-disciplinary team is made up of different professionals. A multi-disciplinary team may work together in a case of child abuse. A social worker, teacher, counsellor, health visitor and the police may work together as a team to support and protect the victim of abuse. A multi-disciplinary team saves time and facilitates sharing of vital information. Cases of child abuse, such as that of Victoria Climbie, where information was not shared, prove the need for a multi-disciplinary approach.

Inter-agency working occurs when representatives from different sectors work together to a common aim. Youth offending services aim to reduce crime and safeguard young people. Representatives from the police, education, probation and health services meet at a strategic level to plan joint working. Inter-agency working is used in cases of domestic violence, where housing officers, the police and social workers share information to support victims. Inter-agency working is encouraged by government policy but there can be problems. For example, not all agencies are equally committed to joint working; not all agencies have enough staff to attend the meetings required for effective inter-agency working.

An example of inter-agency working is the 16+ Care leavers service, which focuses on offering advice, assistance and befriending services to young people aged 16 and above who are either leaving care or who already live independently. This service offers support, accommodation and information about finances, such as grants and benefits. It works closely with specialist agencies in the community, and also with Connexions to provide opportunities for employment/education and training.

Below is another example of inter-agency working, where a housing association works with social services.

Example

Ferngate Project – Birmingham

Ferngate is a Highgate-based accommodation project run in partnership with Trident, a local housing association. Flats are provided for care leavers and support given by both 16+ Careleavers Service and housing support workers.

A four-week assessment period is spent in a training flat at the Project. Referrals are currently made directly to the scheme. Ferngate is one project among a range of accommodation options for care leavers in Birmingham.

ASSESSMENT TOOLS

In order to make sure everything is included in an assessment of needs, or care plan, care workers use a variety of checklists or tools. These might be individually designed checklists or forms, diary notes made by the social care worker, or even diary notes made by service users. Social workers may ask questions and observe. They may use information from networks of those involved or may use the service user's personal history and information from group discussions.

Social workers may even use a flow chart to help them make sense of the variety of information. One of the problems with such a variety of sources is that there may be too much information. It may be all of one type, for example, all about the service user's physical care. Other needs may be missed. Lorraine may be able to express her needs, but not all those in need of an assessment are able to do so.

In an attempt to solve this problem for older people who may have health and social care needs, a single assessment process (SAP) was introduced in the National Service Framework for Older People. (Department of Health, January 2002)

Research tip

The Department of Health website is a useful source of information about the single assessment process.
www.dh.gov.uk/en/Policyandguidance/
Healthandsocialcaretopics/Socialcare/
Singleassessmentprocess/
DH_4015630

The single assessment process is intended to be used across health and social care. It is difficult to share information if there are many different types of assessment tool, so the Department of Health decided to reduce the number approved for care planning. Below is one they have approved to be used in the single assessment process for older people:

Example

STEP (Standardised Assessment of Elderly People in Primary Care in Europe) results from a European partnership to develop evidence-based approaches to assessing older people in primary care. It has been tested in practice settings in the north-west of England and developed with the support of the Royal College of General Practitioners.

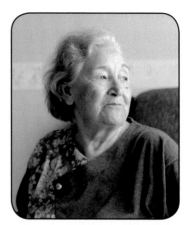

Figure 9.5 STEP is an assessment tool for elderly people.

CASE STUDY: MICHAEL

Michael is 85 years old and lives alone following the death of his wife six months ago. Michael has lived in the house he shared with his wife for the past 50 years. He has no family or friends to help him although a neighbour has been food shopping for him once a week as since his wife's death Michael has found it difficult to leave the house. Michael has difficulty getting up the stairs unaided and since his wife's death he has been sleeping on the sofa downstairs.

Social services are unaware of Michael's predicament because he is frightened that they will put him in a care home if they find out he is struggling to cope in his own home. Michael has been admitted to the nearby hospital on several occasions because he has had a number of falls.

Most of his falls happen when he bends down to turn his fire on. Hospital staff are worried about Michael's ability to cope on his own and say it is not safe for him to return home alone. Michael is very distressed by this and has told the hospital social worker that he must go home or he will kill himself.

QUESTIONS

1. Why might Michael be afraid of going into residential care?

2. Will it be possible for Michael to stay in his own home? If so, what options could Social care workers consider to help make Michael's like at home easier and safer?

Some of the people involved with Michael's care may include:

- a doctor – to check why he is having frequent falls. Perhaps he has low blood pressure or gets dizzy because of an ear infection.

- a nurse – to plan his care during the hospital stay

- an occupational therapist – to assess his ability to cope in hospital and at home

- a physiotherapist – to help with rehabilitation

- a dietician – to look at his nutritional needs

- a nurse from the mental health team – to assess his mental state

- a community matron – to be involved in his care at home.

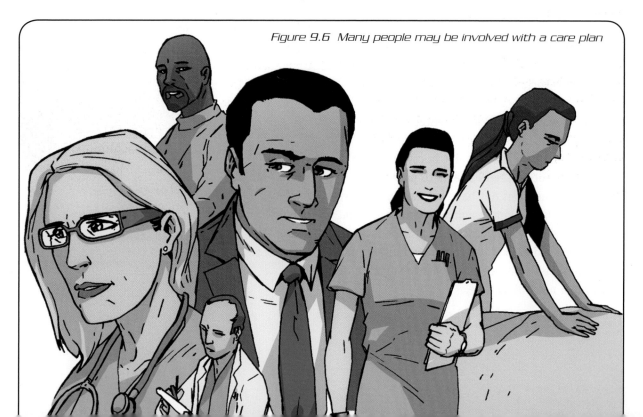

Figure 9.6 Many people may be involved with a care plan

APPROACHES TO IMPLEMENTING CARE PLANS

Behavioural

A behavioural approach to implementing care plans will focus on changing behaviour.

Once a care plan is written it must be implemented or made to happen. This may occur in different ways. For Lorraine, care may need to focus on helping her manage her behaviour. She may need counselling and an anger management course to help her learn to get along with others.

Task-centred

Care may be task-centred. In Michael's situation this may mean that a care assistant is paid to visit Michael at home and help him get washed and dressed. The focus is on the task to be done. Some care agencies allocate time rather than tasks, so Michael may have a carer for an hour. The carer will help Michael to get washed and dressed but will be able to talk to him too.

Research on this topic by Chris Patmore of the Social Policy Research Unit, University of York suggests that there are problems with task-centred services. Care staff are under pressure to meet deadlines and do not have time to chat with clients.

Use of networks

Lorraine and Michael will each need a network of care. Some people have friends, family and neighbours who care and keep contact, but not everyone is fortunate enough to have such a network. Lorraine's father is not in contact with her and her mother seems unable to provide any support. Michael does not have any family support but he does have a kind neighbour who helps him. People who do not have a network of friends and family still need help. This is where voluntary and private organisations can supplement state care in providing a network of care.

> **Think** What organisations are there that might provide support or advice for Michael and for Lorraine?

Use of groups

A variety of groups or organisations can offer help to people in need, as we can see from the examples of Michael and Lorraine.

Example

If Michael goes to his local library he may be able to find out about national organisations such as:

- Cruse – to help him come to terms with his grief and the loss of his wife. There might also be a local branch near him.

- Age Concern –to help him become aware of his rights to stay in his own home

- Help the Aged – for advice about heating costs and care homes if he decides to consider residential care

- Mind – a national charity in England and Wales (with local branches) which works to help people with mental health issues.

Michael may be able to attend locally organised day centres or lunch clubs. His local council and his local library will have a list of what is available.

Research tip

Most areas have a local voluntary services council. In Birmingham the website is www.bvsc.org/ . You can search for a particular service in a particular area – from a befriending service to minor house repairs.

Research tip

In Scotland the Voluntary Health Scotland organisation co-ordinates voluntary health agencies: www.vhscotland.org.uk/library/vol/vol_pub.html

In Northern Ireland the coordinating body is the Department for Social Development Northern Ireland: www.dsdni.gov.uk/index/links/links_govandvol.htm

Example

Lorraine is offered the support of the local Connexions service. Connexions works with people aged 13-19 years and offers advice and information about money, health, careers, work, relationships and many more topics. They even show how to set up a blog!

Lorraine's first priority is to find somewhere to live. A Connexions advisor may be able to advise Lorraine about this and about finding a job to pay the bills. Lorraine has made life difficult by making herself intentionally homeless. Shelter in England and Scotland has local branches and may be able to advise her. Shelter Cymru in Wales and Housing Advice Northern Ireland offer the same service to homeless people.

Use of advocates

Advocacy, where an individual is given support to express their views, is an important way that service users can be heard. UKAN is a federation of advocacy projects, patient's councils, user forums and support groups to help those supporting people with mental health issues. OPAAL, the Older People's Advocacy Alliance UK aims among other things to improve access to advocacy for older people. Michael may benefit from advocacy from either of these organisations.

Lorraine may feel her social worker has not been helpful, or that the housing service has been unfair. The National Youth Advisory Service offers information, advice, advocacy and legal representation to children and young people up to the age of 25, through a network of advocates throughout England and Wales. In Scotland, Children in Scotland works with children and their families, and in Northern Ireland this work is undertaken by Children in Northern Ireland.

The national charities Save the Children, NCH Action for Children, Barnardo's and the NSPCC all work towards promoting the rights of children.

As a result of the Children Act 2004, the Office of the Children's Commissioner was established by Parliament to be an independent organisation looking after the interests and to act as the voice of children and young people. The Commissioner is independent of government, so that it can be impartial. The Commissioner has to work within the framework of the five outcomes described in 'Every Child Matters'(the government's national framework for change) and must follow the United Nations Convention on the Rights of the Child.

Use and abuse of power

Vulnerable people are not confident in asking for their rights. Children, older people, the homeless and the mentally ill, and many others may feel their views are not listened to and they have no power to change things. They may feel they have to accept whatever decisions are made about them. However, legally they have rights. Advocacy empowers vulnerable people and helps them to have a voice in society.

Think How far is it helpful to involve other disciplines and other agencies? Who benefits – the client, the carer, the social worker? Or is it all of them? Can you think of any disadvantages?

KEY PEOPLE

Social worker

Social workers are the key professionals in planning social care. The consultation paper, 'Roles and tasks of social work in England', published by a team from General Social Care Council (GSCC), Social Care Institute for Excellence (SCIE), Children's Workforce Development Council (CWDC), Commission for Social Care Inspection (CSCI) and Skills for Care (SfC) offers this description of good social work:

Example

Good social work:

• Places the service user at the centre of everything it does, concentrates on abilities rather than impairments, balances rights and risks appropriately for children and adults, families and communities, strives for social justice and challenges discrimination and exclusion.

• Carefully uses its legal powers and responsibilities to improve the wellbeing of individuals, families and communities, works creatively within organisational and resource constraints, and is pro-active, preventative, innovative, and creative.

• Takes the lead, coordinating and linking the work of other professionals, family, and carers, to enable people to achieve their potential, strengthen family relationships, support families to stay together, and help vulnerable people to remain living in their own home or in another place they choose.

• Helps people transform and change their lives, putting the focus on problem solving and improvement, and preventing deterioration and breakdown.

• Is evidence-based, uses a wide range of empowering practice, user knowledge and research, and is dedicated to achieving positive change and developing social capital by building safe, strong and caring social networks and communities.

Source: www.gscc.org.uk

Support worker

The term 'support worker' is used to cover a variety of roles. A clinical support worker is a carer in hospital who may have gained an NVQ qualification or may not yet be in trained. Support workers work in a variety of settings in health and social care but are not professionally qualified.

Domiciliary care worker

A domiciliary care worker may be the person to carry out, or implement, the actions required by the care plan. This may involve personal care, such as taking someone to the toilet, bathing them and helping them dress. Some support workers may provide social training care, which may involve taking a client or group of clients on holiday.

Michael may be able to live in his own home if a domiciliary care worker is allocated to help him get dressed in the morning and have breakfast.

Occupational therapist

An occupational therapist will have completed a three year degree at university. The occupational therapist assesses a client's ability to perform everyday tasks such as dressing and preparing a simple meal, and may suggest aids to help maintain independence. Michael may have to be assessed by an occupational therapist to see what help he needs. The social worker would include this in the care plan.

Health visitor

A health visitor is a trained nurse with a post-graduate qualification. The health visitor may also be a qualified midwife. A health visitor or a community matron may visit Michael at home and assess his health needs. Under the single assessment plan, they would already have most of the information they need. His GP (doctor) may refer Michael for a psychiatric assessment and he may then have a community psychiatric nurse.

Lorraine's care plan will focus on her as a care leaver. Her care plan may include sessions with a counsellor, and appointments with a Connexions advisor. This will all be part of the plan of care the social worker organises for her.

We will examine some of these in more detail in the next section, but you can already see how much a social worker has to know in order to do their job!

EVIDENCE ACTIVITY

P1 – P2 – M1 – M2 – D1

For P1 you have to describe the processes of care planning with reference to care planning principles.

Briefly describe a case study of someone needing care. If you base this on someone you know, change the details so that confidentiality is maintained. You can use the checklist below to help you.

Assessing care needs (adapted from Roper Logan and Tierney Model)

	Needs help? Yes or no	Plan for help	Review date
Maintaining a safe environment			
Communicating with others			
Breathing			
Eating and drinking			
Going to the toilet			
Washing and dressing			
Maintaining a stable and safe body temperature			
Mobility			
Work and leisure			
Expressing sexuality or personal identity			
Sleeping			
Death and dying			

Use the case study to assess the person's needs and plan how the needs will be met. You will have to specify how needs are assessed and when the plan will be reviewed and evaluated. This usually happens after 6 weeks but may be sooner if the situation changes.

For M1 you have to explain care planning principles. How do you make sure that the needs, choices and rights of the client are considered? How do you empower the client and put the service user at the centre of this process? Explain how advocates may be involved in care planning. How would you maintain confidentiality?

For P2 you have to identify the importance of multi-disciplinary and inter-agency working on the care planning process. Imagine you are the social worker in this case. What skills do you think you might need when working with Lorraine to produce the first care plan? Make a list and explain why you need each skill. Imagine you are the social worker in Lorraine's case. What other agencies do you think you might need when planning Lorraine's care at 13? Would the same agencies be involved when she is 17? Why is it important to include multidisciplinary and inter-agency working in care planning? Imagine you are the social worker for Michael. What other agencies do you think you might need when planning Michael's care? Why is it important to include multi-disciplinary and inter-agency working in care planning?

For M2 you have to use examples to explain how multidisciplinary and inter-agency working can improve the care planning process.

Here are a few situations to think about:
- Jack is 20 and has learning difficulties. He wants to move out from his parents' home into a place of his own.
- Betty has lived in a small residential home which has to close. She usually attends a day centre twice a week.
- Imran is 12 and in residential care awaiting a foster home. A place may be available soon but it is on the other side of town.

For D1 evaluate the role of multi-disciplinary and inter-agency working in social care.

9.2 Legislation, policy and codes of practice that influence social care practice

LEGISLATION

Legislation, laws or Acts passed by Parliament are legally binding. We also have laws derived from European standards. Laws change and get updated all the time. No one expects you to know all the details of every relevant law but if you work in care you need to be aware of your legal duties and responsibilities.

Research tip

One of the best ways of keeping up to date is to check the relevant government websites such as www.direct.gov.uk and official care sites such as gscc.

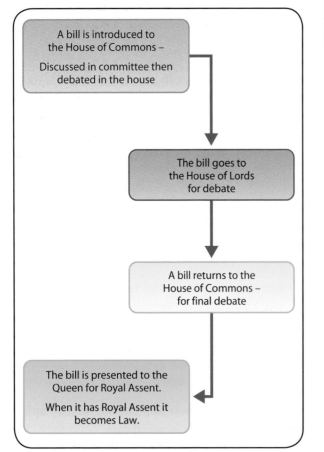

A bill is introduced to the House of Commons –

Discussed in committee then debated in the house

The bill goes to the House of Lords for debate

A bill returns to the House of Commons – for final debate

The bill is presented to the Queen for Royal Assent.

When it has Royal Assent it becomes Law.

Figure 9.7 How a bill becomes law

The Convention on the Rights of the Child 1989

The United Nations office of the High Commissioner for Human Rights (UNHCHR) based in Geneva, Switzerland, adopted the Convention on the Rights of the Child and it came into force in 1990. The United Kingdom has agreed to implement it. All countries who have agreed must report to the Committee on the Rights of the Child (CRC) to say how they are implementing the Convention.

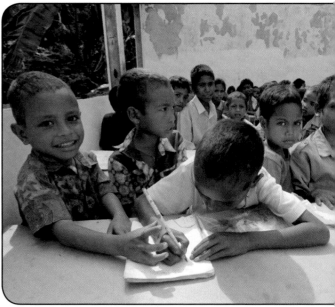

Figure 9.8 The Convention considers the best interests of the child.

Under the terms of the Convention, a child is anyone under the age of 18. The 54 articles in the Convention explain the rights given to children in the countries that have signed the Convention.

The best interests of the child are the first consideration. A child must not be separated from his or her parents against their will unless the courts have said it is in the best interests of the child.

This means that a social worker planning care for a child must make sure the services they offer conform to this standard.

Article 12 of the Convention states that children who are capable of forming a view must be given a voice in any decision that concerns them. Many of the articles form the basis for the Children Act 2004

Research tip

You can read the Convention on the Rights of the Child in full on www.unhchr.ch/html/menu3/b/k2crc.htm

European Convention on Human Rights and Fundamental Freedoms 1950

European legislation covers European countries who have agreed to have these common laws. The European Convention is not global in its scope and differs from the United Nations convention in this respect.

The European Convention on Human Rights and Fundamental Freedoms 1950 has been updated with various protocols to make sure it still applies in the modern world. The latest was protocol 11 in 1998 and gave freedom of assembly.

Research tip

You can read about the European Convention on Human Rights and Fundamental Freedoms on: www.echr.info/

In terms of care planning:

- Article 3 –no one should be subjected to degrading treatment or punishment, so in a care home, people should not be left exposed and naked on a commode while staff make a bed. No child in care should be subjected to degrading punishment.

- Article 4 – no one shall be held in slavery or servitude. Children in foster care cannot be treated as slaves.

- Article 5 – people cannot be detained against their will so no one can be forced into a care home.

Example

You may think conventions such as those described above are unnecessary in a civilized society – unfortunately a recent case study shows why we still need them. In March 2007, Eunice Spry, a foster mother was found guilty of treating her foster children as slaves. She tortured them. The abuse had not been spotted by social workers monitoring the case.

Think Which articles of the European Convention on Human Rights were breached in this case?

Legislation or laws are often revised and changed if they are no longer relevant to society. It is important to use the current version and to put the date of the Act when you write about it.

Health and Safety at Work Act 1974

The Health and Safety at Work Act 1974, also referred to as HASAW (or HSW), is the main piece of legislation covering occupational health and safety in the UK. The Health and Safety Executive is responsible for enforcing the Act and a number of other Acts and Statutory Instruments relevant to the working environment. Care workers must have a safe working environment. A social worker who organises domiciliary care in the service user's own home must make sure that a hoist is available if the service user needs lifting.

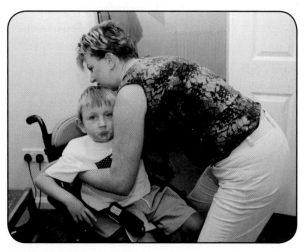

Figure 9.9 It is a legal requirement to protect your back at work

Mental Health Act 1983

This makes provision for the compulsory detention and treatment in hospital of those with mental disorder. The Act is in ten parts and explains when and how a person who is mentally ill may be sectioned or detained in hospital.

Michael, in the earlier case study, would be monitored as he has threatened to kill himself. If his social worker thought Michael was a danger to himself or to others, he might apply for his admission under the civil section of the Act (part2). An approved Social Worker or the nearest relative may apply. Two doctors must recommend the emergency admission. One of the doctors must be approved according to the Mental Health Act. This Act is currently being amended. A new Mental Health Bill is being debated in Parliament in 2007.

The Children Act 1989 and the Children Act 2004

Summary of the Children Act 2004:

Part 1 provides for the establishment of a Children's Commissioner. There will be one each for England, Scotland, Wales and Northern Ireland. Their role is to raise awareness of how children's views are heard and any problems with systems. They will report to Parliament each year.

Part 2 'Children's services in England' establishes a duty on local authorities to make sure there is co-operation and sharing of resources to improve children's well-being. In Lorraine's case, this would mean that the social worker, housing department or housing association and the Connexions advisor must work together, for Lorraine's wellbeing. Local authorities must set up statutory Local Safeguarding Children Boards and key partners must take part. A single Children and Young People's Plan (CYPP) replaces lots of different regulations. Local authorities must have a Director of Children's services and lead member to be responsible for education and children's social service functions, with housing and leisure to be added if needed.

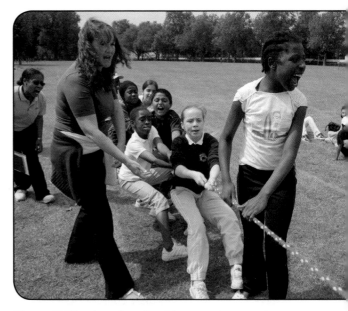

Figure 9.10   Local authorities must promote educational achievement

Inspections must be integrated and there must be Joint Area Reviews. Previously there would be a social services inspection of a nursery, but they did not look at what children learned. Ofsted (education inspectors) looked at what children learned in a nursery school, but did not look at the same things that social services looked at.

Part 5 –'other provisions' includes Section 52, which puts a duty on the Local Authority to promote the educational achievement of 'looked after' children. This will ensure that decisions on placement support better educational achievement. In Lorraine's case this would mean that the social worker who planned her care at 13 must ensure Lorraine can attend school or college, and must support her to do so.

Equal opportunities

Laws about equality include: the Sex Discrimination Act 1975, which states that it is unlawful for an employer to discriminate against you because of your sex.

Age discrimination: from 1 October 2006, there is legal protection against age discrimination. It is no longer lawful for employers to discriminate on grounds of age. This does not apply to services, so Michael can be told he is too old to have physiotherapy!

Research tip

You can find out about your rights on www.direct.gov.uk

Race Relations (Amendment) Act 2000

This Act extends the Race Relations Act 1976 to the police and other public authorities. It is unlawful to discriminate against anyone on grounds of race, colour, nationality (including citizenship), or ethnic or national origin. All racial groups are protected from discrimination. The Commission for Racial Equality oversees the implementation of this Act. A social worker planning care may not discriminate against anyone on racial grounds. Each person is an individual and should be treated as such.

Disability Discrimination Act 1995

This Act gives people with disabilities rights in the areas of employment, education, access to goods, facilities and services and buying or renting land or property. It covers people who have HIV, cancer and multiple sclerosis from the moment they are diagnosed and covers all areas of the public sector.

Example

Michael may be diagnosed as disabled when his falls are investigated. He has a right not to be discriminated against because of this. His social worker may need to bear it in mind when arranging for a home assessment. Michael may need adaptations such as a handrail on the stairs, or a grab rail in the bathroom.

Human Rights Act 1998

This Act came into force in October 2000 and incorporates the European Convention on Human Rights and Fundamental Freedoms into UK law. All public bodies must make sure that everything they do is compatible with the convention rights unless an Act of Parliament makes that impossible. A detailed breakdown of the Convention is given earlier in the chapter. Anyone who believes their Convention rights have been violated can for the first time ask a court in England or Wales to deal with it rather than take the case to Strasbourg, Europe.

Mind, the mental health charity, gives good examples of how this Act may apply. The right to life must be respected. A person threatening suicide must not be ignored. Protection against torture means that clients in care homes must not be tied down to restrain them.

Data Protection Act 1998

This Act came into force on 1 March 2000. According to the Information Commissioner's Office, people have a right to know what is written about them. Information must be kept only for the time necessary. It must be accurate and up to date. People have a right to see what information is held about them whether this is on computer or in paper based records.

Research tip

You can find out more about the Information Commissioner by going to the website: www.ico.gov.uk

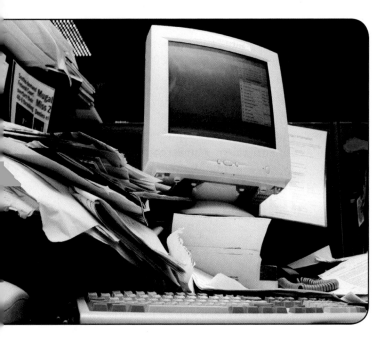

Figure 9.11 Data protection applies to paper-based records as well as computer files

The 1998 Act is different from the 1984 Data Protection Act in some important ways. The Access to Health Records Act 1990 permitted access to manual health records made after November 1991. The Data Protection Act 1998 permits access to all manual health records whenever made, with specified exceptions.

Care Standards Act 2000

This set up the National Care Standards Commission in England and the National Assembly for Wales as the equivalent registration authority in Wales. These bodies can issue minimum standards of care. Local authority fostering and adoption services will be inspected by the Commission and childminding and daycare services for young children will be regulated under this Act, with checks on the suitability of people working with this age group enforced. The functions of the General Social Care Council are set out in this Act. The Commission will keep a list of those unsuitable to work with vulnerable adults and will provide guidance on the charges for local authority homecare services. The Care Standards Act 2000 replaced the Nursing and Residential Care Homes Regulations 1984.

The National Care Standards Commission maintains a register of care homes and domiciliary care agencies. For the first time, local authorities are required to meet the same standard as services in the independent sector. These include care services ranging from residential care homes and nursing homes, children's homes, domiciliary care agencies, fostering agencies and voluntary adoption agencies through to private and voluntary healthcare services (including private hospitals and clinics and private primary care premises).

A General Social Care Council (GSCC) for England, and a Care Council for Wales (CCW), Cyngor Gofal Cymru, regulates the training of social workers and standards in social care through codes of conduct and practice and through other means. These councils maintain a register of social care staff. (The Central Council for Education and Training in Social Work (CCETSW), was abolished by the Care Standards Act 2000)

Inspection and regulation

In England a new arm of Ofsted brings together the regulation of childcare and early years education. Early years education in Wales will continue to be inspected by Her Majesty's Chief Inspector of Education and Training in Wales, through Estyn (the Welsh equivalent of Ofsted).

There is a single list for both England and Wales which is a register of those unsuitable to work with vulnerable adults. Care homes and domiciliary care agencies, prescribed services within the NHS and the independent health sector, and employment agencies and businesses which provide or supply individuals to work in care positions, must refer people to the list in certain circumstances. Care providers must check the list before offering employment to potential recruits in a care position working with vulnerable adults, and must refuse employment in such a position to any person included in the list.

Research tip

You can find out more on www.opsi.gov.uk/acts/en2000/2000en14.htm

CODES OF PRACTICE

Section 62 of the Care Standards Act 2000 requires the General Social Care Council to produce codes of practice for employers and workers and to keep them under review. This includes the General Social Care Council/Care Council for Wales/ Northern Ireland Social Care Council.

The Code of Practice for Employers

In order to meet their responsibilities in relation to regulating the social care workforce, social care employers must:

- make sure people are suitable to enter the workforce and understand their roles and responsibilities;

- have written policies and procedures in place to enable social care workers to meet the General Social Care Council (GSCC) Code of Practice for Social Care Workers;

- provide training and development opportunities to enable social care workers to strengthen and develop their skills and knowledge;

- put in place and implement written policies and procedures to deal with dangerous, discriminatory or exploitative behaviour and practice; and

- promote the GSCC's codes of practice to social care workers, service users and carers and co-operate with the GSCC's proceedings.

Social care workers must:

- protect the rights and promote the interests of service users and carers;

- strive to establish and maintain the trust and confidence of service users and carers;

- promote the independence of service users while protecting them as far as possible from danger or harm;

- respect the rights of service users whilst seeking to ensure that their behaviour does not harm themselves or other people;

- uphold public trust and confidence in social care services; and

- be accountable for the quality of their work and take responsibility for maintaining and improving their knowledge and skills.

Research tip

You can read the codes in full on the General Social Care Council website at www.gscc.org.uk

EVIDENCE ACTIVITY

P3

For P3 you need to use four examples to describe key aspects of legislation, policies and codes of practice that influence social care.

Describe the GSCC codes of practice for employers and the code for care workers. How easy would it be for employers and workers to comply with this code?

POLICY

According to the GSCC code of practice, employers must have policies in place to cover health and safety and equal opportunities. Many employers in care and managing small businesses are unsure how to write a policy. The Health and Safety Executive, a government body, gives the following advice:

Your health and safety policy statement... shows who does what; and when and how they do it.

If you have five or more employees you will need to have a written health and safety policy statement. This should set out how you manage health and safety in your organisation.

You must carry out a risk assessment to identify any risks and then make decisions on how to manage such risks, so far as is reasonably practicable, to comply with health and safety law.

If you employ five or more employees, you must record:

- the significant findings of the assessment; and any group of employees identified by it as being especially at risk.

This would then form part of the general policy of your business on how you deal with health and safety at work and the organisation and arrangements you have for putting that policy into practice.

The policy should be specific to your business, and should be clear about arrangements and organisation for health and safety at work. It should influence all your activities, including the selection of people, equipment and materials, the way work is done and how you design goods and services.

A written statement of the policy and the organisation and arrangements for implementing and monitoring it shows your staff, and anyone else, that hazards have been identified and risks assessed, eliminated or controlled.

When you draw up or review your policy, you should discuss it with your employees or their representatives for health and safety.

Risk assessments

Care establishments usually have more than five employees, so need a health and safety policy. In care there are specific risks, for example, in care homes, a care worker may be exposed to bodily fluids such as urine, vomit, or blood. In a children's residential home, there may be times when children are aggressive. The risks must be assessed before the event happens, and as far as possible the risk should be reduced.

> **Think** What other risks might you need to be aware of in care work?

Employers must:

- have a health and safety policy

- display information about health and safety law or provide each employee with a copy of *Health and safety law: What you should know* (ISBN 0 7176 1702 5)

- have employer's liability insurance

- report injuries.

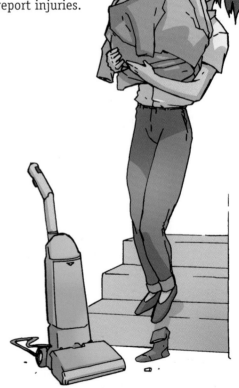

Figure 9.12 Risk assessment aims to stop an accident before it happens

The employer must carry out and record the findings of a risk assessment, looking at the hazard. They must assess the risk. The risk must be eliminated where possible, or reduced if it cannot be eliminated. In a care home, a service user may have difficulty getting to the toilet on time and may accidentally wet the floor. This poses a risk for service users and staff as anyone may slip on a wet floor. A care manager should assess the situation. Has the service user got a urine infection which makes it difficult for them to get to the toilet on time? Do they have other health problems? By considering these issues, the problem may be resolved and the risk of slipping removed. Can the service user be offered help to get to the toilet regularly? Are the floors non-slip? Is there a means of cleaning the floor at once? All these measures will reduce the risk of slipping.

Key words

hazard – anything that can cause harm e.g. chemicals, electricity, working with confused clients
risk – is the chance, high or low, that someone will be harmed by the hazard.

To comply with the requirements of the Health and Safety (First Aid) Regulations 1981 there must be a first aid box available.

To comply with the Reporting of Injuries, Diseases and Dangerous Occurrences Regulations 1995 (RIDDOR) employers must record and report injuries, ill health and dangerous occurrences.

STANDARDS

The Commission for Social Care Inspection (CSCI) registers, inspects and reports on social care services in accordance with statutory regulations and the national minimum standards issued by the Department of Health. Since April 2007 children's services have been inspected by Ofsted.

There are national minimum standards for:

- care homes for older people
- care homes with adult placements

- care homes for adults aged 18-65
- adult placement schemes
- domiciliary care
- nursing agencies.

Some of the standards for Care homes for Older People include information about the choice of home, meal and meal times, privacy and dignity, and the standard and cleanliness of accommodation. Levels of staffing and the management of the home are also covered. A complaints procedure must be in place.

Research tip

You can see these standards on the Department of Health website www.dh.gov.uk/

EVIDENCE ACTIVITY

M3 – D2

For M3 you need to explain the impact of legislation on the concept of care planning.

You may wish to link this to case studies you have already discussed or bring in case studies from placement or journals.

For D2 you need to evaluate the effectiveness of current legislation in promoting care planning and multi-disciplinary/inter-agency working.

'Evaluate' involves a judgement, so how effective is current legislation in promoting care planning and multi-disciplinary/inter-agency working? Give examples to help you evaluate. You may think current legislation is very effective or not very effective, but give examples to support your argument.

9.3 *Values underpinning social care practice*

VALUES

'Values' means principles, or ideals. The values that underpin social care practice vary, according to whose views are heard.

Political

Government, as represented by politicians, have political values. Left-wing political values support the view that care should be free at the point of delivery, from birth through to the end of life. 'Free at the point of delivery' means that people do not pay at the time they receive care, however people do pay for their care through National Insurance contributions. If Michael worked when he was younger, she would have paid National Insurance contributions and so would not expect to pay for his care now. Right-wing political values support the view that we should pay fewer taxes, and save so that we can pay for our care when we need it. Currently, political values are shifting to a more right-wing view of care. People are expected to pay for residential social care if they have more than £16,000 in savings. Costs vary according to the type of care given and the location of the care home, but may be around £500 per week. (Figures approximate for 2007.)

Social

Social values are the values held by society. Again these vary. Society is not all the same. Some people believe we should be responsible for our own care, and that families should care for their own. Others believe that the government should provide care because many families are separated and not all families are in a situation where they can look after their relatives.

> **Think** Who do you think is responsible for looking after the more vulnerable people in our society?

Cultural

Cultural values overlap with social values. In some cultures, it is considered shameful not to look after the older generation. In other cultures, grandparents do not see why they should look after their grandchildren. Lorraine's grandmother may feel that she has raised her own children and now wants time to herself so cannot give Lorraine a home.

Spiritual

Spiritual values may be expressed in terms of religion. Older service users may have spiritual values which help them come to terms with ageing and the end of life.

Moral

Not everyone is religious, but many people have moral values, and have principles of what they consider right or wrong. So, for example, carers may think it is the right thing to do to chat to a lonely service user even if it is not in their job description.

Professional bodies, such as the General Social Care Council (GSCC) and the Nursing and Midwifery Council (NMC), have codes of practice expressing the professional values that those on the register must uphold. Values such as trust, confidentiality and a duty of care are common to social care professions.

CARE VALUE BASE

The care value base is a set of values or beliefs that underpin professional health and social care. The care value base covers five main areas:

* promoting anti-discriminatory practice
* maintaining confidentiality
* promoting and supporting individuals' rights
* acknowledging individuals' personal beliefs and identities
* promoting effective communication.

The care value base is important because it sets out what service users can expect from carers, and it helps carers to be clear what is expected from them. It is incorporated into all health and social care work. A social worker, a care assistant, a health visitor, a nurse and an occupational therapist all work to the same care value base. Their codes of practice may be worded differently, but the values are the same.

Policies and charters are based on the values too. 'Choose and Book' is a policy which allows patients to choose their hospital or clinic and book an appointment with a specialist. This links to promoting and supporting individual rights. The Patient Advice and Liaison Service (PALS), set up by the Department of health, acts on behalf of their service users when handling patient and family concerns. They liaise with staff, managers and organisations, to negotiate solutions and improve the way that services are delivered.

Research tip

You can find out more by going to PALS Online. See www.pals.nhs.uk/

All care professionals have a responsibility to reflect on and monitor their own practice to ensure they apply the care value base in their work.

INDIVIDUAL RIGHTS

All people have rights, as we have seen in the Human Rights Act. Everyone has a right to be respected, treated equally and not discriminated against. Lorraine had the right to a home and was found one by the housing department. Others had a right to a safe environment, so Lorraine had to be evicted to protect them from harm.

Example

Michael wants to be treated as an individual and not just put in a home. He is entitled to his view and has the right to be heard, to be treated as an individual in a dignified way; and allowed to live in the privacy of his own home. Michael has a right to be cared for in a way that meets his needs and he is entitled to an assessment of his needs under the Care Standards Act 2000.

Example

Lorraine too has rights. She is now a care leaver. She has been given a home but had to be evicted because her behaviour was a risk to others. Service users have the right to see information about them. Under the Data Protection Act they have a right to get changed any information which is incorrect. Lorraine might feel that her case has been unfairly represented and that she was not to blame for the quarrels in her previous housing. She might have been bullied. If she sees her case notes, she may wish to challenge the accuracy and the judgment that she is intentionally homeless. Lorraine may not be able to express her views in professional language but she has a right to use her preferred language.

Service users who have hearing impairment may use sign language. Service users who have limited or no English have a right to be cared for in a way that meets their needs. It should not be assumed that a speaker of Welsh knows English.

WORKER'S RESPONSIBILITIES

Provision of Active Support to enable service users to communicate their needs

Care workers have a duty to provide active support to enable patients and service users to communicate their needs, views and preferences. A care worker who works in a Welsh speaking area may need to learn some Welsh in order to support service users appropriately. A care worker working with a deaf client may need to learn sign language. Communication is a basic skill required in caring. If the carer cannot communicate with the service user, they may not be able to offer choice or represent their client's views.

While it is unrealistic to expect carers to learn every language in a diverse community, there is a responsibility to communicate with service users. Sometimes the tension between rights and responsibilities proves difficult in practice. Carers have limited time to learn languages, but common sense can be applied. A carer may already speak Welsh or use sign language, and so may be the appropriate person to help other carers gain some of these skills when caring for a particular client who has these needs.

Filing correctly and securely

Care workers must comply with the Data Protection Act 1998 mentioned earlier (see page 29). The Information Commissioner's office provides a checklist to guide those involved with recording. The social worker helping Lorraine must make sure that case notes are securely stored, are accurate and up to date. Records must be readable and dated. Written records must be signed. Electronic records must be securely stored so that no one can hack into a system and download personal information about others.

9.4 *Ethical principles in relation to social care*

ETHICAL PRINCIPLES

Definition of ethics

One definition of 'ethics' is 'the study of moral standards and how they affect conduct'. Ethical principles are concerned with the honourable way to behave in life.

Role in social care

Ethical principles are important in social care because care workers are working with vulnerable people who could easily be exploited. Therefore there is a moral obligation to maintain particular standards to protect those who are in need of care.

Duty and protection, independence; autonomy

Care workers have a duty to protect service users from harm, while at the same time helping them to develop independence and autonomy. A care worker with no moral principles could easily take advantage of vulnerable service users such as Michael or Lorraine.

MORAL STATUS (VALUE OF LIFE)

Reasons for ethical considerations

Ethical or moral principles enable good care to happen. They are essential values which should be inherent in every carer. People without ethical principles should not work in care. One of the reasons the GSCC set up a register of carers is to make sure those without ethical principles are not allowed to work with vulnerable people. In 2006 a social worker was removed from the register for having an inappropriate relationship with a service user. Another social worker was cautioned for failing to disclose convictions for thefts. One was removed from the register, which means they cannot work as a social worker, for sending and receiving several emails from his work email account containing offensive, discriminatory and obscene content.

Research tip

Look at this website for more information on the need for ethical principles: www.gscc.org.uk/ News+and+events/Media+releases

SITUATIONS CARE WORKERS MAY FACE

Conflict of interest

Often in care situations, there can be conflicts of interest. There may be disagreements between the service user and an organisation; for example, when Lorraine quarrelled with her house mates, this was in conflict with what the housing department wanted. Sometimes there can be conflict between service users and other service users – Lorraine and her house mates could not get along.

Service users can disagree with their relatives and friends. For example, Lorraine was also in conflict with her mother.

Sometimes there is conflict between service users and workers; for example, Michael wanted to be discharged home, but the hospital staff felt he would not be able to cope. Care work is never easy. Sometimes there are difficult decisions to be made and the carer may not always agree with the service user's choice.

Example

Lorraine's social worker must have been disappointed that Lorraine was evicted.

Michael's social worker may have been concerned that Michael would not be able to manage even with all the support in place.

However it is not the role of the care worker to make decisions for service users unless they are legally appointed to do so in a situation when a service user is deemed to be mentally incapacitated.

Rights and duties, obligations

The care worker's duty and obligation is to provide help and information so the service user can make an informed choice.

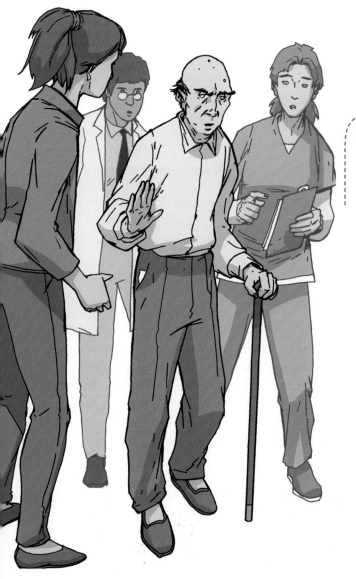

Figure 9.13 It is never easy being a carer

Choices of individuals

If Michael's health check up showed that his falls were due to a terminal illness, the care worker must abide by any decision Michael makes about who can be told. If Michael's neighbour asks, a care worker must not disclose information. The care worker must direct the neighbour to speak to Michael. Confidentiality must not be breached.

Sometimes, however, it may be necessary to breach confidentiality. If Michael goes back home and becomes depressed, he may think of suicide again. He may tell her carer that he is thinking of ending it all. In such a situation, Michael is a risk to himself, and the carer must report this to her manager even if Michael asks her not to.

One of the most difficult situations for a carer is when a service user who is ill asks the carer if they are going to die. Any service user who is ill should be given information about their condition, but this is usually the job of the doctor.

Example

Michael's carer may know that Michael has an incurable illness but, when asked outright, 'Am I going to die?' may not know how to respond. In such circumstances it is better to get the doctor or nurse to talk to Michael. It is inevitable that we are all going to die at some time, but Michael may want to know how long he has left, which is a different matter.

Sometimes people with a supposedly incurable illness do get better or live much longer than expected; while others may seem to give up and die quickly. There are appropriate ways of giving such information and sometimes a carer may need to refer a service user to someone else in the care team.

Majority versus minority

Carers may be faced with a situation where they suspect abuse. It is possible that Michael was being financially abused by relatives or friends. He may be neglecting himself and not eating. He may have bruises where another carer has roughly treated him. Lorraine has been sexually abused in the past and as a vulnerable young person may be easily exploited again. Her key worker may suspect that Lorraine is being abused.

Telling the truth

These are clear cut situations where the carer or key worker must tell the truth and report their suspicions. They are often the only people who can help stop the abuse. The situation is difficult if the suspected abuser is a co-worker, but the carer has a legal obligation or duty of care to the service user and so must report concerns. This can be difficult for the carer as they may feel in a minority and may not always get the support they would hope for from other workers.

Rationing services and resources

In the current political climate, where care is increasingly rationed, and resources are not available, carers may face difficult situations.

Example

A carer who is sent to a client's home alone when it is a two-person visit may be unable to give the care needed. A carer in a residential home may work a 14-hour shift and get home only to be called in again because of staff shortages. These carers are torn between wanting to make sure clients are cared for and maintaining safe practice.

Just think what could go wrong. The domiciliary carer who tries to lift a client alone without a hoist may injure themselves and the service user. The care assistant who works for 14 hours followed by another 6 hours may make a mistake with medication, or get short tempered with a service user who is incontinent. Working long hours and working in understaffed situations can lead to accidents or worse. Carers working in such situations must raise the issue with their line manager and record their concerns. If matters do not improve, and managers seem unable to provide the staffing levels or resources needed, the Commission for Social Care Inspection has an online alert form to report concerns under 'safeguarding adults'. The report can be made anonymously.

We are now in a situation where good practice is more clearly supported. The social care workforce is being trained to provide a high quality service where values are embedded in the planning and delivery of social care. In some areas, resources are scarce but this means we must make efficient use of the ones we have. Planning cuts down accidents, reduces complaints and in the end costs less, which means we can spend more on what really matters – good quality care.

EVIDENCE ACTIVITY

P4 –P5 – M4

For P4 you must describe the values that underpin social care practice.

For P5 you need to describe ethical principles in relation to social care.

For M4 you must explain the roles of individuals and organisations in relation to values and ethical practice.

Prepare an induction booklet to explain to a new carer the values that underpin social care practice and ethical principles in relation to social care. Include a section which explains the roles of individuals and organisations in relation to values and ethical practice. Choose a social care organisation such as a residential care home and refer to guidelines from the General Social Care Council.

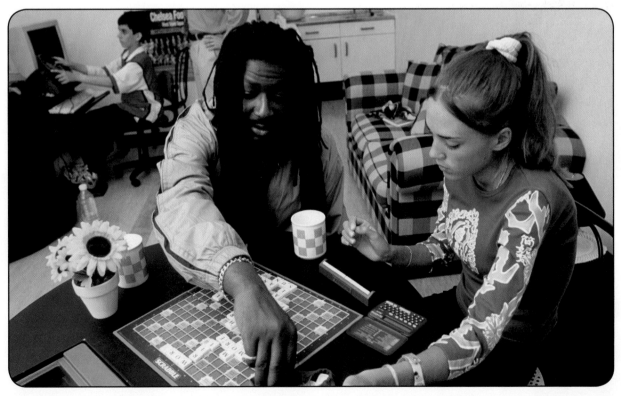

Figure 9.14 Resources are sometimes stretched but good quality care is the aim

Supporting and Protecting Adults

unit 11

In this unit you will learn about the differing needs of people using health and social care services and how to develop supportive relationships which respect individual rights. You will also learn how such relationships may be abused. This involves a study of types of abuse, indicators of abuse and the potential for abuse in health and social care services. You will look at the factors which make people vulnerable and at the practices developed to minimise abuse.

The topics dealt with in this unit are sensitive. For some people, issues of abuse can be emotionally upsetting. It is important that you have access to support services such as counselling if any of these issues affect you. Your tutor should be able to arrange this in confidence.

It is strongly recommended that this unit is studied in the later stages of the course, so that you will have developed more understanding of professional work and will have had some experience of work placements. You may also have gained some knowledge and understanding of protection issues during work experience which will help you understand the issues better.

Learning outcomes

On completion of this unit you will:

So, you want to be an...

Occupational Therapist

My name Ben Lucas
Age 26
Income £24,000

If you are looking for a job that can change people's quality of life for the better then read on. This exciting and varied role could be just the job for you.

What do you do?

I help people with physical, mental health or social problems to lead as independent a life as possible. My clients have problems resulting from accidents, operations, illness and ageing. I assess the need for specialist equipment and home adaptations to enable patients to live as independently as possible. I work with people recovering from stroke and head injuries as well as post operative patients and patients with physical disabilities. I work with a team of other professionals and with the patient and their family.

How did you get into the job?

I have a B.Sc. (Hons) degree in Occupational Therapy. My degree was mostly based on theory but about one third was supervised fieldwork placements. Previous experience of working with older people or people with mental health issues is a real advantage. Some of my colleagues have a Foundation degree in Health and Social Care.

What skills do you need?

You need good people skills and an ability to inspire confidence in patients. You must be able to build good working relationships with other professionals and be able to build a relationship with patients. You need to be very organized and be able to manage your time effectively. You also need to be able to get along with people from all walks of life.

> " **It's great to know you are making a real difference to people's lives** "

What's the pay like?

Pretty good. New Occupational Therapists (OTs) earn £19,000 to £24,000, more if they move on to specialist posts. Consultant OTs earn up to £50,000.

What are the hours like?

Usually 9 to 5 although occasionally I will have to work later into the evening.

What are your plans for the future?

I would like to stay where I am at the moment, I really enjoy being part of a team and the daily contact with clients is very rewarding; it's great to know you are making a real difference to people's lives. Eventually I would like to become a consultant OT but I have a lot to learn before then.

Grading criteria

The table shows what you need to do to gain a pass, merit or distinction in this part of the qualification. Make sure you refer back to it when you are completing work so you can judge whether you are meeting the criteria and what you need to do to fill in gaps in your knowledge or experience.

In this unit there are three evidence activities that give you an opportunity to demonstrate your achievement of the grading criteria

page 52	P1, M1 and D1
page 59	P2, P3, P4, and M2
page 69	P5, P6, M3 and D2

To achieve a pass grade the evidence must show that the learner is able to...	To achieve a merit grade the evidence must show that, in addition to the pass criteria, the learner is able to...	To achieve a distinction grade the evidence must show that, in addition to the pass and merit criteria, the learner is able to...
P1 Explain how individual rights can be respected in a supportive relationship	**M1** Explain how supportive relationships can enhance the life experiences of individuals receiving health and social care services	**D1** Use examples to evaluate the role of supportive relationships in enhancing the life experiences of individuals receiving health and social care services
P2 Describe different forms of abuse that may be experienced by vulnerable adults		
P3 Describe different indicators of abuse in vulnerable adults		
P4 Describe the potential for abuse in health and social care contexts	**M2** Analyse the potential for abuse in four health and social care contexts	
P5 Describe strategies and working practices used to minimise abuse		
P6 Identify the legislation, policies and procedures that protect adults receiving health and social care services.	**M3** Explain how legislation, policies and procedures contribute to the protection of vulnerable adults.	**D2** Analyse the role of multi-agency working in minimising the risks of abuse in health and social care contexts.

11.1 *Developing supportive relationships with adult users of health and social care services*

Before we get into details, let's look at what is required. Important words here are relationship and adult users.

SUPPORTIVE

In health care, people who use the service are called 'patients'. In social care they are called 'service users' or 'clients'. In this unit, we will use all these terms but remember that these terms for people who use the health and social care services are jargon. Sometimes jargon can hide the fact that they are people first and foremost.

The word supportive tells us something of the type of relationship or bond we are hoping to build. It is the kind of relationship which encourages a person to develop their abilities and achieve their potential.

The type of relationship in health and social care is specified. It must be supportive which means helpful. An adult user of health and social care services is a grown up and mature person who uses these services. So this section could be called 'Know how to develop helping connections or bonds with grown up mature people who use health and social care services'.

But things are not so straightforward. Some adults who use health and social care services are not necessarily mature, for a variety of reasons. People with some types of learning disabilities can be physically 'grown-up' in years, but may not have developed mentally. Someone with autism may take everything literally at face value. If you say 'let's jump to it' that is what they may do – jump! They may find it difficult to understand why you are talking about jumping when you really mean 'Let's be quick'. An older person with dementia may not behave in an 'adult' way because dementia affects memory. They may forget where they are and who they are with, and behave inappropriately.

There may be cultural reasons why an adult does not behave in the way you might expect. In some cultures, older people order younger people around and this can seem very rude. They may not say 'please' or 'thank you' because it is not part of their culture and there are no words for 'please' or 'thank you' in their own language. Different social customs can be confusing for anyone. In western cultures, it is good manners to shake hands when introduced but some adults do not like to be touched. They may be from a different culture where touching is very bad manners and people bow instead.

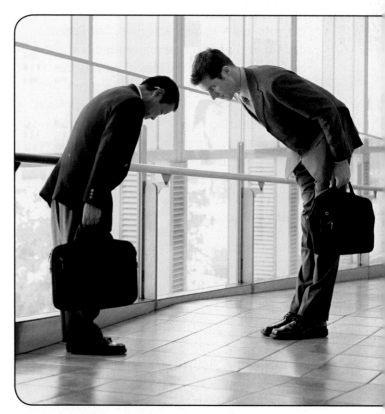

Figure 11.1 Different cultures greet people in different ways

It is important to remember that adults are individuals. Each person is unique. In order to develop a supportive relationship with someone, you first have to get to know them. One final point, this unit is about supportive relationships with adults – not with children. Issues of abuse are very relevant when working with children and young people but the focus of this unit is about adults.

> **Think** What different cultures are you aware of? Think of some cultural differences you know about. How might that knowledge help you when developing a supportive relationship with someone from another country?

Humanistic approach

This is based on the humanistic school of psychology. Abraham Maslow and Carl Rogers were two main theorists of this school. Maslow suggested that all humans have a hierarchy of needs which start with basic survival needs. Once these needs are fulfilled, we seek love and belonging. The respect of others and our own increasing self esteem then enable us to develop our potential – to 'self- actualise'. Carl Rogers developed the idea of person-centred or client-centred counselling. The idea of putting the client at the heart of what we do as carers stems from Rogers' work. A humanistic approach looks forward, starting from where the client is now. It does not try to explain why a person has those behaviours, but tries to help them establish more effective ways of behaving. There is more on these theories in Unit 8, Psychological Perspectives in Health and Social Care.

A humanistic approach uses the values of:

- unconditional positive regard

- empathy

- genuineness.

'Unconditional positive regard' means that the carer regards the person positively, and is looking for the best in them. 'Unconditional' means without conditions. This is better explained by looking at the opposite – conditional regard. A parent who says to a child, 'I won't love you if you do that' is putting conditions on the relationship. A parent who says to a child 'I will always love you – whatever you do,' is unconditional in their love. 'Unconditional positive regard' means the carer accepts the person as they are, without conditions, and looks for the best in them. 'Empathy' means 'seeing a situation from another person's viewpoint'. It is not sympathy, feeling sorry for someone, but it is about trying to understand them. 'Genuineness' is about being open and honest, not pretending.

A carer using the humanistic approach would start by establishing the relationship on a person-centred basis. A good way to do this is by listening to and informally observing the person. What are they saying? Do they seem to mean what they say or do their actions contradict their words?

> **Think** Have you ever heard a tired and angry parent say of their child 'I'll kill him!'? Do you think they mean it? What do you think they really mean?

The focus would be on establishing a relationship where the client felt safe, reassured and trusted the carer. Part of establishing a relationship is about setting clear boundaries. Relationships take time so the carer would not hurry a client but if they have time limit, for example an hour for a visit to a client's home, the carer would say so and say when they would have the next meeting.

If a carer has established a non-judgmental and accepting approach, the person may misinterpret this. People with few social skills might think the carer's friendliness is flirting. A carer must let the client know that this support is part of their professional work so that the client has a clear understanding of the relationship being established.

CASE STUDY: HOSPITAL EMERGENCY

Mrs A went to hospital as an emergency with a suspected stroke. She was 75 years old and was the main carer for her husband, who was left at home. She had weakness down the left side of her body and was admitted to a ward for observation. The nurse on the ward made Mrs A welcome and settled her down in a side room, helping Mrs A into a nightgown. She offered to help unpack but Mrs A rudely told her to leave things alone and stop prying.

Instead of unpacking for her, the nurse asked Mrs A what she could do to help. Mrs A told her to bring a telephone. When the phone arrived, Mrs A told the nurse to leave it and go away. The nurse did so, but made sure she could see Mrs A through the glass in case she had another stroke. She knew that helping Mrs A contact her husband was the most important thing she could do at that time. By enabling Mrs A to continue her caring role for her husband, she was in fact helping Mrs A to keep control of her life.

Mrs A was used to doing things for herself and looking after her husband. The possibility of a stroke frightened her because she was worried about who would care for her husband. Having access to a telephone meant she could make arrangements for a friend to stay a few days and care for Mr A.

QUESTIONS

1. What reasons could there be for Mrs A's rudeness?

Helping and enabling

A supportive relationship is one which is helping and enabling - helping the person to gain skills and enabling them to take control of their own life.

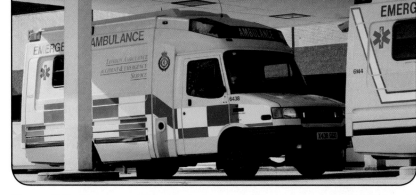

Figure 11.2 Clients in A&E should be given choices where possible

Empowering, giving choices

'Empowering' means 'giving power'. Empowering clients means giving power to clients. The nurse looking after Mrs A could have said, 'I'll make the call for you – just give me the details.' This would have taken power away from Mrs A and she would have been dependent on when the nurse could make the call. Mrs A would have been anxiously waiting to know if friends could stay and care for her husband. By giving Mrs A the phone the nurse was empowering her, giving her the chance to make choices about who to ring, when to ring, what to ask them to do. A supportive relationship does not take away from what a patient can do. It supports them in developing skills, such as coping with change.

Maintaining privacy

Privacy or time alone is valued differently by different people. There are cultural differences – some cultures traditionally have lots of people around all the time and people with these cultural values may be lonely if put in a side room alone. For others, visitors and other patients are not what they need when they are ill. A side room is their ideal situation.

> **Think** What aspects of privacy are important to you?

A carer should find out what a patient prefers and try to maintain the level of privacy the patient wants, balanced against care requirements. Mrs A might want to be left alone to sleep, but if she has a stroke caused by bleeding in the brain (an intracranial bleed) she may drift from sleep to unconsciousness. The nurse may have to check Mrs A every 15 minutes, but should explain why this is done.

Like the rest of us, most users of health and social care services value privacy for personal care such as bathing, dressing or undressing and going to the toilet. A supportive carer will find out what the patient prefers and try to maintain the desired levels of privacy. This could vary from individual to individual. For one client it might mean leaving the toilet door unlocked because they are frightened they might be ill and need help. Another client may want to be left alone until they ring for help.

Mixed sex wards raise issues for patients and carers alike. Mrs A might have to move into a six-bed bay, opposite an elderly confused gentleman who keeps shouting and undressing. The nurse would check with Mrs A how she felt about the mixed sex bay and explore possibilities of moving beds or using screens to maintain as much privacy as possible.

> **Think** How might you feel if you were ill and had to spend a few days and nights on a hospital ward with male and female patients? What help would you expect from the nurse in maintaining your privacy?

Maintaining confidentiality

Confidentiality refers to privacy of information. Mrs A may be offered a social worker before she is sent home. The social worker will be able to get some of the information such as address and telephone number from joint care plans, but some information may not be recorded. Mrs A may be entitled to help if she has less than £16,000 in savings. The social worker may therefore have to ask detailed questions about personal matters.

In a supportive relationship, the social worker will be sensitive to the needs of the client and sensitive to the legal duty to maintain confidentiality. For this reason, he or she may ask personal questions in a private room where no one can overhear what is said. Of course, the social worker must also be careful not to leave the notes lying around on the nurse's station where anyone can read them. You can read more about confidentiality in Units 1 and 2.

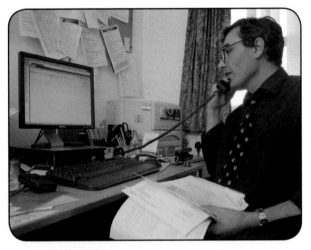

Figure 11.5 Confidentiality of information is an essential part of a supportive relationship

Where there is a supportive relationship, a patient may feel able to tell the nurse everything on their mind. At times this can be difficult. The nurse must always be aware that if the client discloses anything which is a risk to the client themselves or to others, the nurse must break confidence and report it. Perhaps Mrs A has cared for her husband for many years and at times felt unable to cope. She might even have thought of ending it all for both of them with an overdose of sleeping tablets. If she tells this to the nurse, then the nurse must report this as Mrs A's mental situation is a threat to both her life and her husband's life. The nurse has a moral obligation to warn Mrs A of the circumstances when she has a legal duty to break confidentiality. This can threaten the supportive relationship as the nurse then does not have the full trust of the patient.

Advocacy

In a supportive relationship, the nurse or social worker puts the client at the centre of what is done. But not all service users are able to express their views clearly. This is where advocacy is useful. Advocacy may be informal or formal. Informal advocates may be volunteers who have an understanding of the client's views and can express their views clearly.

> **Key words**
>
> advocacy – support, backing, to give active verbal support

An advocate may speak on behalf of a client, for example at a case conference where a client's care is reviewed. Check Units 1 and 2 for more information about advocacy.

> **Research tip**
>
> In some areas, Age Concern offers advocacy services. You can find out more on www.ageconcern.org.uk

Promoting rights

In supportive care relationships, the rights of individuals are promoted by the carer. A patient has rights to a good standard of care and to a clean environment with trained staff, and these are rights which many nurses promote on a daily basis. The carer has a duty of care to promote the statutory or legal rights of the client to anti-discriminatory service, to confidentiality and to respect. Sometimes the carer may need to draw the attention of managers to shortfalls in these areas.

Non-judgemental

Non-judgemental means 'not judging'. Carers must not judge clients. No one can really know what drives others to addiction, aggression, abuse, criminal or other destructive behaviours. There is a saying that, if you want to understand a person, you should walk a mile in their shoes. A supportive relationship is about empathy or understanding; not judging someone involves just that.

Some carers find this a difficult idea but it is not really so hard. Care values and human rights both uphold respect for life. The behaviour is not the person. It is possible to like a person but not like what they do. It is possible to support a person but not support what they do. For example, a starving person may steal a loaf of bread. A non-judgmental approach will try to see the situation from the individual's viewpoint in order to understand them. This does not mean that the carer approves of stealing.

> **Think** Is there anyone you might find it difficult to care for? How would you care for that person if you had to do it?

RELATIONSHIPS

In the case study about Mrs A we saw a relationship that promotes the views, preferences and independence of individuals and key people. Mrs A wanted to remain as a carer for her husband. He, as a key person, wanted to stay at home.

> **Think** Identify a relationship from your placement experience where the views, preferences and independence of individuals and key people were promoted. You may be able to identify a time when you did this in the caring role. This could be used for Unit 6 evidence of your personal and professional development.

In the case study about Mrs A the relationship supported Mrs A's communication of her needs. The humanistic psychologist Abraham Maslow (see page 44 and Unit 8) suggested we have basic physical needs which must be met first. Many care plans are based around these needs, in the form of activities of daily living. They include needs for food and fluid, personal hygiene, elimination. Higher level needs include safety needs, a need for love and belonging and for self esteem.

Example

Let's consider the way the nurse in the case study supported Mrs A in communicating her needs and preferences.

- She asked Mrs A what help she needed.

- She did not take it personally when Mrs A was rude.

- She did not retaliate when Mrs A was rude.

- Her body language was probably open, otherwise Mrs A would not have requested the telephone.

- She listened and responded to Mrs A's request even though it was not expressed politely.

Think What is the difference between needs and preferences?

Needs are things we cannot live without. We have a basic need for food. However, preferences are about choice. We need food, but that need may be fulfilled by giving, for example, porridge or toast at breakfast. Some people have a preference for toast while others prefer porridge. Either of these choices would meet the need, but only one would meet the person's preference.

Differences between family, friends, professionals

In all relationships there are differences. Differences are normal. Life would be very boring if we all liked the same things, dressed the same way and had the same thoughts. The important issue is how we handle differences.

In health and social care, service users can be vulnerable and open to abuse by others. When a person needs the health and social care services, they need help. A relationship is established between the professional and the client or patient but often the patient has family and friends who may also wish to be involved. Differences may arise. See what might happen in Mrs A's case.

CASE STUDY: MRS A's FAMILY AND FRIENDS

Mrs A has a married daughter, Sally, who lives on the other side of the country and has a busy job. Sally is very worried about her parents. She knows Mr A's health is poor and that her mother does all the caring. Sally thinks it would be better if her mum and dad went into sheltered accommodation in a warden-controlled flat. Then they would have someone to call if things went wrong. She rings the ward and asks to speak to the nurse looking after Mrs A. She explains her views and asks the nurse to arrange this accommodation for her parents.

Mr and Mrs A have a neighbour, Maryam, a young woman who works as a carer at the local residential home. Maryam is the person who stays with Mr A while his wife is in hospital. She told Mr A what had happened but Mr A became quite aggressive and kept shouting for his wife. He had forgotten what Maryam had told him. Maryam realised that Mr A needed a lot of care. She wondered if Mrs A would be able to cope with him much longer. When Maryam rang the hospital to ask after Mrs A, she had a quiet word with the nurse and suggested that Mr and Mrs A would be better going into the residential home where she worked. They would both be safe and looked after all the time.

Mrs A wants to get back home. Sally wants her parents to move into sheltered accommodation. Maryam, the neighbour, wants Mr and Mrs A to move into residential care. A supportive relationship puts the patient at the centre of care. The nurse must give Mrs A full information about all the options and let the patient choose.

Relationships between equals – caregiver/care receiver

The relationship between care giver and care receiver is one of equals. This means that neither is more powerful than the other. In the past, service users were seen as less powerful. Doctors, nurses and social workers told clients what was good for them and carried that out. People with learning disabilities were sent to live in institutions because the doctor said so. A doctor might tell a patient that they must have an operation, or move to a healthier climate, and the patient agreed. This has now changed. Doctors and nurses advise. The patient decides whether they will have the treatment offered. Most patients do follow professional advice because professionals have more information and experience, but the old-fashioned relationship of subservience and unequal power balance has largely gone.

Key words

subservience – sub means below and servience comes from the same word for service. Subservience means being willing to give in to the will of another.

Power and subservience

Before 1945, health care and social care were only available to those who could afford them. If you were ill, you had to pay to see a doctor. Most doctors, nurses and social workers belonged to the middle class. They were used to telling servants what to do, and to having power over others. The working classes were usually poor and grateful for any help they could get from health or social care professionals. Some working-class people were used to working as servants for the middle class and so were subservient.

Research tip

The Victorian Web is a good resource if you want to know more about how health and care developed. See the website www.victorianweb.org/

Health visitors would visit poor people in slum housing and tell them how look after their children. Social workers distributed charity, and the recipients had to be grateful for this. The patronising attitude of telling people what was good for them was embedded in the origins of health and social care services. In 1846, wealthy people donated blankets which were lent out for a fee, to poor people who could not afford to buy their own. Organised Blanket Lending societies were one of the many ways that rich people could feel good about helping poor people. They did not think of it as belittling poor people. They thought they were doing their duty. Belittling means making fun of, or mocking someone (making a person feel small). Some people think that care professionals will belittle them if they are honest about their needs and that health and social care workers are patronising, and intend only to make clients feel inferior.

Key words

Patronising – treat in a condescending or demeaning way

Think How would a care professional make sure that the client knows they are not patronising them? How would a care professional make sure the client knows they will not be belittled?

DEVELOPMENT OF RELATIONSHIPS

Communication and body language

Relationships are established, developed and sustained through communication. In Unit 1 communications are explained in detail, but you will probably remember that most communication is non-verbal. Your body language – how you stand or sit, how you place your hands, whether you cross your legs – all send out messages to other people. Facial expressions can be friendly or frightening. This is why we use them in emoticons. Look at these emoticons (pictures for expressing emotions) and try to work out what emotions they are expressing.

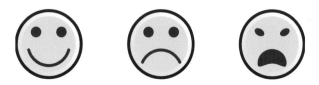

Figure 11.4 What emotions are being expressed here?

A patient will decide within a few seconds whether they trust the care professional enough to talk openly with them.

Touch

Touch can be used to express communication but must be used carefully to avoid misunderstanding. Putting an arm round a client is a powerful gesture which should be avoided. It puts the carer in a position of power and disempowers the client. Touch is not used in counselling situations and is best avoided in developing relationships.

Key words

disempower – to take power away, making someone powerless

Sometimes touch is unavoidable, for example, when a carer has to help a client with washing or dressing or other personal care, but touch should only done with the client's permission and for a specific purpose.

Research tip

You can read about the meaning of touch in care work in an article by Julia Twigg (1997) called 'Bathing and the Politics of Care' in Social Policy & Administration 31 (1), 61–72

Think Would you tell a person your hopes and fears if you did not trust them?

Trust

Trust, the belief that the carer has the client's interests at heart, is essential for the development of care relationships.

Other aspects of trust include:

- reliability - being able to depend on someone

- consistency of approach – being the same each time

- fairness - showing justice and equality

- objectivity – not letting personal problems or dealings with other people affect your own attitude towards the individual requiring care.

Think Can you find examples of any of these aspects of trust in the relationship between Mrs A and the nurse?

The final point about being objective – not letting personal problems or dealings with other people affect your own attitude towards the individual requiring care – is very important. When we react to our feelings and emotions we are behaving subjectively. This is fine at home and when with friends. It is not acceptable at work. Professional practice, which you study in Unit 6, demands that we put our personal views to one side when dealing with clients. We must be objective, treating everyone equally.

Nurse C may have had an argument with his girlfriend before coming on duty, and he may be angry. Would you expect him to speak angrily to patients on the ward? Definitely not! A professional must put personal feelings on one side in order to care for everyone equally. Social worker D may have been mugged by a group of young boys. Would you expect this to influence her attitude to every young male who is a client? Definitely not!

Part of being a care professional is that you can work objectively. Care professionals care for humanity and do not discriminate. This is why in a war zone, anyone who is injured, whether ally or enemy, is given health care.

INDIVIDUAL RIGHTS

Much of this is already covered in depth in Unit 2 which covers equality, diversity and rights in health and social care. This section will therefore touch briefly on the topics. Individual rights are set out in the European Convention on Human Rights 1950, the later Human Rights Act 1998, Data Protection Act 1998 and the Freedom of Information Act 2000. We also have equal opportunities legislation and policies on equal rights. Procedures, which are guidelines about how to do something, are derived from these policies.

When developing relationships in health and social care, all rights must be upheld. This is not so difficult if you treat the person as an individual in a dignified way. The right to be respected, treated equally and not discriminated against is enshrined in law.

Example

The right to dignity: at the outpatient's clinic, a large lady is given a gown but it does not cover her. The nurse offers her an extra gown to slip her arms into, so that she is decently covered.

The right to be protected from danger and harm: Sam has learning difficulties and has not yet travelled on the bus alone. He wants to go home from the day centre alone but the support worker suggests it would be better for him to do the travel training programme first.

The right to be allowed access to information about themselves: service users have a right to see the information that is held about them and to have any inaccurate information changed.

CASE STUDY: HOME FROM HOME?

K is of Pakistani origin but was born and educated in this country. He has never been to Pakistan – in fact he has never been outside England. K suffers from kidney failure and is waiting for a transplant. He needs regular dialysis to stay alive. As he arrives at the dialysis unit one day he overhears two new carers talking about foreigners who 'ought to be sent back home'. He is astonished to hear his name mentioned as one of them.

QUESTIONS

1. Which of these rights have the carers ignored?

- to communicate using their preferred methods of communication and language
- to be treated as an individual
- to be respected
- to be treated equally
- not to be discriminated against
- privacy
- protection from harm and danger
- data protection
- diversity.

2. What impact would the carer's words have on developing a supportive relationship with this client?

Communication

Clients must be able to communicate using their preferred methods of communication and language; cared for in a way that meets their needs, takes account of their choices and protects them. Sam uses BSL. When he sees the GP, he has to bring in a signer because the GP does not understand BSL. Sam has lost his right to privacy if he wants to communicate. How could this be avoided? Perhaps Sam could write down what he wanted to tell the doctor. But he would not then be communicating in his preferred method.

Diversity and differences

Care relationships must support diversity and differences in culture, religion, race, disability, sexuality, beliefs, and behaviour, eating and hygiene habits.

Example

Poppy, a carer at Meadowsweet Care Home is on her break and pops down to the local chip shop. In the staff room, she eats the chips out of the paper, using her fingers. When her early lunch break is over, it is time to serve the residents their lunch. They are having rice and chicken. It is Mrs Begum's favourite meal of the week. When she was a child in Bangladesh, she had chicken curry on special occasions. Everyone in her country ate with their right hand making sure the gravy never went below the middle of the fingers. As she settled herself down at the dining table, she regretted the fact that she had to use a knife and fork. The food just didn't taste as good.

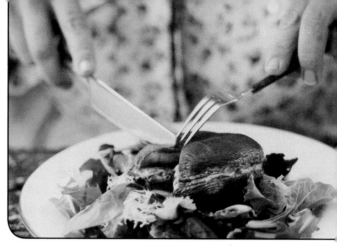

Figure 11.5 Eating habits are bound up with culture

> **Think** To what extent does Meadowsweet Care Home support cultural diversity? Could anything else be done to develop a supportive relationship with this client?

EVIDENCE ACTIVITY 1

P1, M1, D1

You should base this assignment on a case study from one of your placements with adults. You may be able to link this to Unit 6 Personal and Professional Development in Health and Social Care. Of course, you must ensure confidentiality so you will not name the person. Call them 'A' or give them a different name. If you have not been in placement yet, think of a case study from a television series.

For P1 you need to explain how individual rights can be respected in a supportive relationship.

For M1 you should explain how supportive relationships can enhance the life experiences of individuals receiving health and social care services.

For D1 you should use examples to evaluate the role of supportive relationships in enhancing the life experiences of individuals receiving health and social care services.

You may need more than one case study to cover a variety of rights. For P1 you will need to say what rights there are and how they can be respected. M1 develops this by asking how supportive relationships can enhance or improve life experiences. You may be able to give examples of supportive relationships enabling choice, or supporting rights to respect. The distinction point requires evaluation. Look at the strengths and weaknesses of the relationships you considered in M1.

11.2 *Types of abuse and indicators of abuse in health and social care contexts*

TYPES OF ABUSE

> **Key words**
>
> abuse – to ill treat

As carers we work with vulnerable clients who are unable to defend themselves. This is why they need care. Unfortunately abuse does happen. For this reason we must be aware of how to recognise it. The table below lists types of abuse and gives examples.

Table 11.1

Type of abuse	Examples
Physical	Hitting, slapping, rough handling, misuse of medication, misuse of restraint
Sexual	Coercing an individual into participating in an act which they have not or cannot give consent to, inappropriate touching
Psychological	Threats, humiliation, bullying
Financial	Theft of money/possessions, misuse of a service user's benefits
Neglect	Not meeting an individual's care and health needs, e.g. physical, emotional, social, cultural, intellectual and spiritual
Discriminatory	Mistreatment e.g. due to ethnicity, gender, age, disability, sexuality, health status, religion
Institutional	Abuse and/or poor practice throughout the organisation, through organisational procedures
Self-harm	Self-inflicted wounds, drugs, alcohol, medication
Domestic violence/abuse	Physical, sexual, psychological

> **Research tip**
>
> Action on Elder Abuse (AE) works to protect older adults. Find out more at www.elderabuse.org.uk

Some of the examples are obvious but a few need explanations.

Physical abuse

This happens when clients are physically hurt. Sometimes service users become a risk to themselves and to others. On these occasions, if the client seems to be about to hurt themselves, they will be restrained for their own good. Restraint is a specific technique designed to minimise the risk to clients and to carers. Restraint does not involve hitting the client or sitting on their chest. This is misuse of restraint.

Sexual abuse

Sexual abuse includes coercing an individual into participating in an act which they have not or cannot give consent to.

> **Key words**
>
> coerce –force, persuade or bully

Some people with mental health issues or learning disabilities may be particularly vulnerable to sexual abuse. Someone who is fully aware of what is happening will be assertive enough to say no or report the incident. People struggling with low self esteem or those who are not socially and emotionally mature may lack the capacity to make an informed choice. Capacity in this situation has a specific legal meaning.

Psychological abuse

This bullying behaviour can include name calling and humiliation. It may mean isolating someone from contact with others, either by leaving them alone for long periods of time, or by putting them in a place where they are unable to communicate with others. Putting a client to bed at 8pm to get her out of the way is psychological abuse.

Financial abuse

Financial abuse can happen anywhere. A carer may 'borrow' money from a resident and forget to pay it back, or a relative may visit and persuade granny to change her will in their favour.

Discriminatory abuse/neglect

This can happen if a client's needs are repeatedly not met. For example, a Catholic resident may wish to see a priest, but only the Church of England vicar visits, and no one passes on her request to the local Roman Catholic Church. Obviously it also involves physical neglect if a service user's health and care needs are not met.

> **Example**
>
> Mr X may be denied a place in a residential home because he is only 50, despite the fact that he has advanced early dementia.

Institutional abuse

Institutional abuse can occur by default – it happens because no one thinks it is their responsibility to do anything about it. When carers say 'we always do it that way' or 'that's the way the manager wants it done', they are not looking at a situation from a client's viewpoint. Erving Goffman studied asylums and found that total institutions put the needs of the institution before the needs of patients. Examples of institutional abuse include: putting all the residents to bed before the night staff arrive to ease their work load; making all residents get up at the same time so the day staff can do breakfasts; not offering choice because it saves time.

> **Think** What routines are there in your placement? Whose needs are met by these routines – the needs of the clients? The needs of the staff? The needs of the management?

Self-harm

Abuse may be self-inflicted. A client may eat too much or too little, or eat something they know is harmful for them; for example, a diabetic client might eat sweets. Sometimes a person who is mentally ill may cut themselves as away of coping with their feelings. Others may become addicted to drugs or alcohol.

Domestic abuse

Domestic abuse may be in the form of physical or sexual violence; or it may occur in subtle forms of psychological abuse which undermine a person's self esteem.

INDICATORS OF ABUSE AND SELF-HARM

Abuse and self harm may not be detected for some time. Carers should be suspicious if any of the following indicators appear.

Inappropriate injuries/bruising

These may include such problems as repeated fractures. Rib fractures may occur if someone is kicked or punched.

Inappropriate bruising, i.e. not caused by an accident or fall, may typically include black eyes, if someone has been hit in the face, or defensive bruising on arms if someone has put their arms up to protect themselves.

Burns and scalds

Burns can be an indication of abuse, such as cigarette burns on the body where an abuser has stubbed out cigarettes on the victim.

Scalding can be an indicator, particularly of the lower body and feet, if someone has been put into a scalding hot bath, or scalding of the mouth and chest if forced to drink a very hot drink which spills onto the chest.

Malnourishment

People who are malnourished may have pressure sores on hips and shoulders. Skin does not heal because they have insufficient vitamin intake. There may be sores at the corner of the mouth due to lack of vitamin C. The patient may have a sore tongue due to lack of vitamin B. They may be listless and lack energy due to insufficient carbohydrate intake. They may be dehydrated – skin and lips are dry and cracked. Malnourishment may be self inflicted or it may happen as a result of neglect in hospital.

Research tip

Age Concern has a national campaign called 'Hungry to be Heard', which aims to end the scandal of malnourishment in hospitals. For more information see www.ageconcern.org.uk

Low self-esteem

Poor hygiene and lack of self care can show that a person thinks little of themselves. Sometimes people are excessively well dressed and appear to take a lot of time on self-care, but they are doing so in order to please someone else. Celebrities often have low self-esteem. They do not value themselves but rely on the opinion of others to affirm their self worth. When fashion turns against them and fans drop away, the celebrity may have a crisis as they have never learned to value themselves through their own eyes.

Emotional withdrawal

This happens when a person becomes uncaring of what happens to them. They show no emotions. They have trusted and been betrayed by those who should have protected them. They no longer know who to trust so give up trying to engage with the world and instead withdraw into themselves. Erving Goffman describes the inmate role, where a resident stops trying to fight for individuality, and comes to an acceptance that they do not matter.

These indicators show a failure of care. It may be failure of systems but ultimately it is a failure of carers to care. It is a cause for concern that abuse occurs and a cause for shame that the most vulnerable people who seek help are let down by those who should help them.

11.3 Understand the potential for abuse in health and social care contexts

> **Think** So how does it happen? How do caring people become so uncaring?

CONTEXTS

In the home

women's aid
until women & children are safe
www.womensaid.org.uk

Figure 11.6 National domestic violence charity Women's Aid Federation of England

Abuse happens in the home, in the community, in residential care, and in institutional care, wherever there are relationships involving power. In the home where nobody sees except perhaps the children, one partner may have more power than the other. In a loving relationship this power is used to help the other person. When the relationship is not loving, the power is turned against the weaker partner and the situation becomes abusive. Power comes from money, knowledge and status in our society. Power also comes from a person being bigger or stronger than another; they can be physically stronger or mentally stronger. Abuse is misuse of this power.

Domestic abuse is not just abuse of women by men. Women experiance 89% of domestic abuse, some men are abused by their wives but do not ask for help because they are ashamed, especially as this is a society where men have traditionally held more power than women. Abuse can occur in homosexual and lesbian relationships as well as heterosexual relationships.

In the community

In the community abuse can occur where a dominant group abuses an individual or a minority. Homeless people may be beaten up, robbed or raped by members of the community. Homeless people often have other problems. They may have drug or alcohol addictions, be mentally ill or may have run away from an abusive partner or parent. There is no safety on the streets. Homeless people are even more vulnerable because they are not visible. People walk past doorways and turn away rather than make eye contact with a homeless drunk or a spaced-out junkie. Mainstream care services rarely stretch as far as the homeless. GPs are reluctant to take homeless people as patients because they are expensive, especially if they have a drug habit. Social workers are reluctant to work with homeless people because they are part of a transient population, moving on as soon as anything has been arranged for them. The homeless get little help.

Residential and institutional care

In residential care, abuse can happen on a personal level, perhaps from one resident to another, or from one resident towards a carer, or from a carer towards residents.

In institutional abuse, the power of the organisation may be brought to bear on a 'difficult' client, who may have sold his or her home to come into care, and may have no way out. Care home residents are often trapped due to lack of economic power. Care workers too lack power. They are among the lowest paid workers in the country. Many care workers leave the caring role, unhappy with the standard of care but unable to do anything as they need a reference in order to move out to a different job.

Under the new Mental Health Bill going through Parliament in 2007, there is a hotly debated clause about detaining people against their will. The government wants to detain people with untreatable personality disorders. Many people think this is an abuse of human rights.

> **Think** Should we lock up people, who have done nothing wrong, if we cannot treat their personality disorder?

Health and social care contexts provide the setting for abuse but abuse does not happen in every health and social care context. The potential must be there – combined with predisposing factors. It is a bit like explosives. There is a fuse, the gunpowder and a lighted match but they must come together for something to happen.

Key words

potential – possibility

POTENTIAL

The potential for abuse happens when there is:

- bullying within care services
- invasion of privacy
- abuse by carers
- system abuse
- abuse by service users
- abuse of carers.

Bullying may happen between clients, between carers and from client to carer, and even carer to client. See if you can spot the bullying incidents in the following case study.

CASE STUDY: BULLYING IN THE CARE HOME

Poppydene Care Home is a fairly happy place; residents get on well and help each other with the crossword and with bingo. Unfortunately there is a bully among them called Fred. He comes into the lounge, ignores the friendly smiles and stomps across to an empty seat next to Maggie, who is deaf. When Maggie gets up to go to the toilet, he tries to trip her up with his walking stick. When she comes back to her seat, he starts swearing at her and calling her names. Maggie gets scared and looks anxiously round for the care staff.

Rose, a care assistant, comes to Maggie's rescue and helps her to another chair at the far end of the lounge. Fred swears at Rose and later, when she takes him a cup of tea, he throws it over her. Rose thinks she ought to report the situation to the manager. But Rose is rather scared to do this as her manager is a bit of a bully herself, and can often belittle staff in front of clients, relatives and other carers. Nevertheless, Rose plucks up her courage, knocks on the office door and goes in to report the incident.

As she thought, her manager was not sympathetic. In fact she blamed Rose for the whole incident and said that Rose must have tripped and spilled the tea. She even told Rose she would stop the money for the broken tea cup from her wages.

Rose wasn't sure this was legal, but she didn't say anything. She needed the job and the extra hours with her growing family to feed.

Later that shift, Rose took Maggie to the bathroom, then upstairs for a nap. As she settled down, Maggie reached for Rose's hand and said 'Thank you nurse, you are so kind – not like the other one who's on at night. She takes me to the toilet and leaves the door open so she can keep an eye on me while she turns down the bed. That's it then. I'm in for the night. It's a long time from half past eight at night until they get you up next morning but she won't let me have a call bell and won't let me go to the toilet. She shouts at me if I wet the bed but I can't help it.'

Rose knew that all this was wrong. Residents should be able to go to the toilet, and have a call bell. They should be treated with dignity too, and not left exposed on the toilet. Rose knew she ought to report this to the manager, but with a sinking heart realised that the night carer was the manager's daughter. Rose knew nothing would be done. Perhaps she should ring the Care Standards Commission Inspectorate, but she really needed the money from her job.

On the way home she bought a paper and started looking for a new job.

In this case study there is bullying within care services, in a residential care home. But unfortunately bullying can occur in a client's own home or in hospital too.

Invasion of privacy happens when carers forget that a residential home is the client's home. They should knock before entering a client's room. Not many people would like to be on public view when sitting on the toilet. The carer should respect Maggie's right to privacy.

In this case study, abuse by carers happens with the night carer abusing Maggie. But in addition to this, Rose's manager is abusing her power as a care home manager in threatening Rose and in not taking note of potential abuse.

System abuse is shown by the routine which is designed to fit the needs of the staff rota, not the needs of the client. How many people would choose to go to bed at 8.30 every night? A system which is not designed to offer choice is potentially an abusive system.

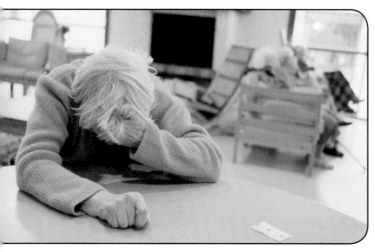

Figure 11.7 Abuse in care homes is a serious issue

Abuse by service users is shown in Fred's treatment of Rose and of Maggie. Unfortunately this is not a rare situation. As older people live longer, some develop dementia, but there are not enough specialist care homes with specially trained staff to meet demand. Sometimes a social worker has to make an emergency placement, when relatives can no longer cope. If there are no places in a specialist unit, and a care home has a bed free, the client will be put into ordinary care accommodation. This was the situation with Fred, who was waiting for a place in a specialist unit.

He was aggressive and abusive to staff and other residents because of his dementia. In the case study there is abuse of carers from Fred, because of his dementia.

Remember, bullying within care services is not confined to residential care. It can happen in day centres, drop-in centres, clinics and hostels. Bullying is harassment. Sadly, the potential for bullying is everywhere – wherever people interact. In health and social care we interact more often with people, therefore the possibility for bullying is greater.

PREDISPOSING FACTORS

Factors which make abuse more likely to happen include:

- learning disabilities

- mental health issues

- age

- dementia

- previous history of having been abused.

Learning disabilities

Learning disabilities in themselves do not predispose a person to being abused; but rather it is passive acceptance of whatever happens which makes them more likely to be abused. People with learning disabilities may not know their rights. If they have been in the care system for a long time, they may be used to doing what they are advised to do, rather than making their own decisions.

Mental health issues

When people have mental health issues they are not always able to see things clearly. Someone who is depressed may feel the world is a dark place and there is no point in trying to do anything, so they do not try to fight abuse. They may have low self esteem and feel that they must be in the wrong; it is all their fault. This can happen when an abuser is plausible and skilled in abusing.

Age

Look back at Unit 8 and Erikson's theory of life stages. As a person ages, they may feel isolated and despairing. They may welcome any contact with people, even if the relationship is abusive, rather than be alone.

Dementia

Dementia is a condition characterised by memory loss. As a person develops dementia they may forget the names of family and friends. Many older couples care for each other and as dementia develops they struggle to cope. A husband may care for his wife, but she no longer recognises him. She may become aggressive towards him and even fail to recognise her own grown-up children when they visit. Caring for a person with dementia on a full-time basis is very demanding physically and emotionally. Carers need a lot of support but sometimes this support is not available. When things get really bad, a husband or wife may lose control and hit the person they are caring for. Dementia is a predisposing factor for abuse because there is not enough support in place for carers.

Previous history of having been abused

When someone is abused, they may think it is their own fault. A man or woman who has been the victim of domestic violence may get little sympathy and people may even say that they must have done something to deserve it. If someone has been abused and not had support such as counselling to work through the situation, they may have low self esteem. An abuser recognises someone with low self esteem and may target them as being vulnerable.

> **Think** Think of an example of bullying or abuse. It may be something you remember from school, or it may be an example from a television series. Was the person who was abused passive and accepting about what happened to them?

EVIDENCE ACTIVITY

P2 – P3 – P4 – M2

For P2 you need to describe different forms of abuse that may be experienced by vulnerable adults.

For P3 you have to describe different indicators of abuse in vulnerable adults.

For P4 you have to describe the potential for abuse in health and social care contexts.

For M2 you need to analyse the potential for abuse in four health and social care contexts.

You should write an assignment to cover P2, P3, P4, and M2. You can either use a case study from a television programme or use the case study of Maggie (page 57). You will need to add more details to Maggie's case study to cover the requirements for P2 and P3.

M2 requires four contexts; you might use a day centre, a residential care home, a hospital, a supported housing scheme, a mental health unit, a drop-in centre or a support group. You may think of other health and social care contexts. If you wish to describe the potential in four contexts for P4, you can use the same four in M2 but remember to analyse the potential.

11.4 *Understand working strategies to minimise abuse*

There are several strategies to minimise or reduce the risk of abuse. Some are broad strategies such as laws and regulations. Some are more detailed and specific, such as policies relating to different organisations. The Care Standards Act 2000 reorganised the regulation of social care, establishing a framework to protect vulnerable people. It established the National Care Standards Commission (NCSC). The Act introduced strategies such as the Protection of Vulnerable Adults (POVA) scheme.

Key words

strategies – plural of strategy, a plan or a way of doing something

STRATEGIES

Protection of Vulnerable Adults Scheme (POVA)

The POVA Scheme was introduced in the Care Standards Act 2000. The scheme establishes a list of people who have been banned from working with vulnerable adults aged 18 years and over. This is known as the POVA list. It covers England and Wales, and covers care workers in care and nursing homes, including agency workers, care workers for domiciliary care agencies, and adult placement carers. These workers must have Criminal Record Bureau (CRB) clearance plus they must be checked against the POVA list before they can start work in care. In this way, people who have been banned from caring for vulnerable people will not be employed again in such jobs.

Research tip

You can read more about POVA on the Department of Health website. Look under publications and search for POVA: www.dh.gov.uk

Care Homes Regulation

The Care Homes Regulations 2001 were amended in 2003 as the Care Homes (Amendment No. 2) Regulations 2003 but were originally outlined in the Care Standards Act 2000. The Care Homes regulations set out who may be considered a fit person to manage a care home, how information on fees should be given to people, and what checks should be made on employees to make sure they are suitable to work with vulnerable people. The Care Homes regulations are designed to protect vulnerable clients from abuse, especially financial abuse.

National Service framework

National Service Frameworks (NSFs) are strategies for improving specific areas of care. They set goals which are timed and measured and were set out in the NHS Plan 2000 and in 'Saving Lives: Our Healthier Nation'. There are NSFs for many areas but perhaps the NSFs for older people and for mental health are most relevant to this unit.

The NSF for older people, published in 2001, sets standards for the care of all older people. It covers home care, residential and hospital care. In a ten-year plan this NSF aims to get rid of age discrimination, ensure care is coordinated and specifically looks at stroke, falls and mental health problems associated with older age.

The NSF for mental health looks at the mental health needs of adults up to the age of 65. It looks at tackling the discrimination and social exclusion experienced by those with mental health problems and reducing the suicide rate in this group of people. According to the Department of Health: 'At any one time around one in six people of working age have a mental health problem, most often anxiety or depression. One person in 250 will have a psychotic illness such as schizophrenia or bipolar affective disorder (manic depression).'

Multi-agency working

This involves agencies working together. The NSF for mental health looks at multi-agency working. Most people with mental health problems are cared for by their GP with the primary care team, but some people with metal health problems need care from several agencies working together to provide housing, training and jobs. MIND, the leading mental health charity in England and Wales, is actually a federation of local mental health charities. They provide services from campaigning and advocacy through to support housing.

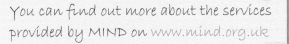

Research tip

You can find out more about the services provided by MIND on www.mind.org.uk

Partnership with service users

MIND works in partnership with service users and promotes their views. In their campaign for better black and minority ethnic mental health services, MIND called for information, translation and interpreting services, and training for mental health staff so that service users can be treated equally. MIND works with professionals and service users to provide information and training for volunteers and professionals, and to influence purchasing decisions to provide accessible rural mental health services. Giving people with mental health issues a voice will help to reduce the potential for abuse.

In the NSF for older people, one of the aims is to improve joint working between professionals and within organisations. A single assessment process has been developed to aid decision-making processes. Nurses and social workers share the same paperwork, thus reducing the potential for hidden abuse.

Forums such as local branches of MIND or Age Concern empower service users by giving them a voice to influence organisational policies and training. MIND has already identified the need for cultural awareness in multi-agency working with people with mental health issues.

WORKING PRACTICES

Working practices can prevent abuse by effective:

- needs assessment
- care planning cycle
- person-centred practices
- written and oral communications
- use of IT in sharing information between professionals
- anti-oppressive practice
- anti-discriminatory practice.

Needs assessment

Needs assessment may include what a person says as well as what they leave unsaid. This may sound a bit odd, but think of a person who has been in an abusive situation. When asked what they need, they may be afraid to say because they no longer trust anyone. They may just say, 'I'm OK – I don't need anything. Just leave me alone.' They may be depressed and have a low sense of their own worth. They may need counselling, but might not say they need it because they do not know such as service exists. Effective needs assessment looks at the whole person.

Care planning cycle

An effective planning cycle helps to prevent abuse. Just because someone has had their needs assessed does not mean they are protected from abuse, indeed sometimes this is when abuse starts. Eunice Spry, a foster carer, abused the children in her care and was convicted in 2007. Only an effective planning cycle which monitors care and conducts reviews with service users in confidence can reduce the potential for harm. In the Spry case, the children were too afraid to say what was happening and the social workers did not check up after complaints were received.

Research tip

You can find out about the Eunice Spry abuse case by looking at the following source: www.gloucestershire.police.uk/news/1841.html

Person-centred practices

Person-centred practices reduce the potential for abuse by giving the service user a voice and giving them power. One effective scheme which empowers clients and reduces the potential for abuse is the Direct Payments scheme. This is where service users are given the money to employ their own carers, rather than social services arranging carers for them. In effect the service user employs the carer directly, reversing the traditional power balance. When a client employs the carer, they have the power to change their carer if they do not like them.

Written and oral communications

Written and oral communications reduce the potential for abuse by improving communication between care professionals. Consider the case of a child admitted to casualty with multiple fractures and the scars of old burns. The nurse or doctor examining the child must contact a social worker at once to inform them that the child might be the victim of physical abuse. It could be that the child is already known to social services and is at risk. By communicating and sharing information between professionals, abuse can be reduced.

Example

The case of Victoria Climbie illustrates this. Victoria was looked after by her aunt and her aunt's boyfriend. They starved and beat her, made her sleep in the bath and tied her in a black plastic sack. She died aged 8 years old with 128 injuries to her body. Throughout her case she had been seen by professionals at hospital, by the social services and had also been seen by a pastor. They did not communicate with each other, and the pattern of abuse went undetected. The Laming Report recommends one simplified document and a 'common language' for use across all agencies. It specifies the information that must be recorded and arrangement for sharing this information. If communication had been shared, Victoria Climbie would have been alive today, instead of a statistic.

The government developed 'Every Child Matters', a strategy for joint working to make sure such abuse does not happen again.

Research tip

You can read the story of Victoria Climbie in the report represented by Lord Laming to Parliament. Follow the link and click on Report. www.victoria-climbie-inquiry.org.uk

IT

The use of IT in sharing information between professionals is as yet in early stages. The computerisation of the NHS is proving more difficult than first thought, and there is a heavy reliance on paper-based records in health and social care. When the system is developed, it will become an effective way to communicate between professionals, but as yet there are unanswered questions about the confidentiality of information which make this problematic.

Anti-oppressive practice

Anti-oppressive practice means empowering the patient or service user. As people have more power, there is less chance of them being abused. Every private care home must publish a guide to pricing and there must be a complaints procedure. In health services, patients are empowered by having access to information. 'Choose and Book', an initiative to help people choose when they will have their first outpatient's appointment, is an example of giving patients power.

Research tip

Find out more about 'Choose and Book' on www.chooseandbook.nhs.uk/

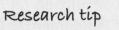

Anti-discriminatory practice

Anti-discriminatory practice involves treating each person as an individual. This approach reduces abuse as it looks at the whole person, and does not stereotype. Training on anti-discriminatory practice is now part of every professional's training in health and social care. A person may be gay, a carer for elderly parents and a recovering alcoholic. Previously some care professionals would have seen the person's homosexuality as a key aspect to be addressed and would have planned to meet these needs or would have discriminated against them on the grounds of sexuality. Either way is poor practice. A person is a complex mixture of attributes and only they can say what they feel is most important to them. Anti-discriminatory practice accepts people for what they are.

PROCEDURES FOR PROTECTION

Procedures are guidelines for how to behave. Each organisation has a protection procedure, often in the form of a flow chart. Policies are general statements on how the organisation approaches a situation. POVA (see page 60) is an organisational policy. The system of first checks is a procedure.

Organisational policies and procedures

The Social Care Institute for Excellence (SCIE) gives a procedure for how to report abuse. They suggest the following:

1. Call the police and the local adult protection officer if you think a crime has been committed or if there is a risk of harm.

2. If you are not sure that it is abuse, contact the local authority adult protection coordinator.

3. If there is no risk of immediate harm contact:

• The commission for Social Care Inspection for care homes (including nursing homes), domiciliary care services or adult placement schemes, or raise your concerns with the service, or the funding authority.

• With NHS services, raise your concerns with the service or with the primary care trust (PCT) providing the service.

Once suspected abuse is reported each area has multi-agency adult protection procedures which they must follow.

Research tip

You can find out more about the work of the Social Care Institute for Excellence by looking at their website: www.scie.org.uk

Lines of reporting include who to contact. In a care home the procedure might be as shown in the case study below.

CASE STUDY: LINES OF REPORTING

Rose at Poppydene Care Home is helping Maggie to get changed. She notices bruising on her back and arms. Nothing was said at handover, and there is nothing in Maggie's care plan about this. Rose documents her findings on the care plan and reports her finding to the senior person on duty, who then informs the manager who contacts social services. Rose does not gossip about this to others because it would breach confidentiality. She reports it and also records it in full, with a date and signature, because written records provide evidence which may be used in a court of law. Bruising may indicate abuse but this may not be abuse. It might be a health problem. Service users have the right to freedom from abuse – therefore Rose has to follow procedure.

Example

Think back to the previous cases study with Rose, when Maggie disclosed that the night carer shouted at her and would not let her use the toilet. Rose should report the situation and record the event in the care plan, following the procedure. The actions to take in the event of disclosure are the same as for suspected abuse. Maggie might feel upset and worried that someone was going to get into trouble. An advocate, an independent person who supports the client, might be useful here. The local advocacy service would provide an advocate for Maggie.

Think At your work placement – find out what the policy says on abuse. What is the procedure for reporting abuse? What actions should a person take if they suspect abuse? Who do they report to? What happens when they have reported suspected abuse?

LEGISLATION

There is a lot of legislation designed to minimise abuse. Sometimes these laws are repealed or changed as further laws are introduced.

Research tip

A good way to keep up to date is to use the government website to find out what is new: www.direct.gov.uk

Think When researching on the Internet, do you really need to read a whole Act? Look for the short executive summary which sums it all up.

European Convention on Human Rights and Fundamental Freedoms 1950

This sets out certain human rights for people if their country has signed up to the Convention. Article 3 forbids degrading or inhuman treatment or punishment. Tying someone down to keep them quiet, or shouting at them because they have wet the bed would breach article 3 of this convention. The Human Rights Act 1998 incorporates the European Convention into English law.

Sexual Offences Act 1976

The Sexual Offences Act 1976 was amended by the Sexual Offences Act 2003. In this Act, rape is redefined to include penetration of the mouth. Penetration by an object is now an offence. Previously people have been acquitted of sexual abuse because they knew the legal loopholes. Now the law is stricter and includes more categories of sexual abuse. This should act as a deterrent to would-be abusers.

Mental Health Act 1983

Part 2 of the Act specifies who can be forcibly admitted into care, and the procedure for doing so. The Act minimises the risk of people being detained when they do not need to be, as two doctors have to agree that the patient is suffering from a mental disorder that requires hospital admission and that the person should be detained in their own interests or safety, or to protect others. Part 4 of this act specifies who can be treated against their will. Clear guidelines such as these minimise the risk of abuse and unlawful detention.

A new Mental Health Bill is being debated in Parliament and Codes of Practice will be introduced.

Mental Capacity Act 2005

The Mental Capacity Act 2005 section 1 sets out five principles which support the idea that everyone has the capacity and the right to make their own decisions. People have the right to support to enable them to make their own decisions even if they seem to be unwise decisions. People who do not have capacity must have decisions made for them which have their best interests at heart. This law gives legal support to client's rights.

Care Standards Act 2000

The Nursing and Residential Care Homes Regulations 1984 and sections of the 1989 Children Act were repealed by the Care Standards Act 2000 which brought children's homes, independent hospitals, nursing homes and residential care homes under one item of legislation. Part 7 deals with the protection of children and vulnerable adults and sets out the POVA regulations for those working in care.

'No Secrets: Guidance On Developing and Implementing Multi-Agency Policies and Procedures to Protect Vulnerable Adults from Abuse', published in 2000 by the Department of Health and the Home Office, gives guidance to local agencies that have a responsibility to investigate and take action when abuse is reported. By working together across sectors such as health, social care, housing, justice and education to share information and coordinate responses, abuse will be reduced.

Speaking Up for Justice is a scheme which ensures that vulnerable or intimidated witnesses are provided with special measures to enable them to give their best evidence in court. Special measures may include giving evidence from another room by a live television link or using video evidence in cross examination. A 'vulnerable witness' is someone under 17 years old or someone who because of mental disorder, significant impairment of intelligence or social functioning or physical disability or disorder may be unable to give evidence in a the usual court room. An 'intimidated witness' is a person who may be frightened or distressed about giving evidence. Abuse is minimised if an abuser knows they may face justice and they will not be able to intimidate their victim.

Example

Action on Elder Abuse is one example of how the increased role of the voluntary sector has helped expose and reduce abuse in care homes. NACRO provides housing as well as advice to help with the resettlement of offenders.

Research tip

Find out more about Action on Elder Abuse – www.elderabuse.org.uk/ and about NACRO – www.nacro.org.uk

NHS and Community Care Act

The NHS and Community Care Act 1990 established the purchaser/provider split in care and gave a greater role to the independent and voluntary sectors. Many of the charities which support patients' rights have gained a larger role under this Act either as care providers themselves or as advocates for patient's rights.

The expanding role of the independent sector provides alternatives to statutory care. Domiciliary care agencies enable people to have the choice to stay in their own home. As people have more choice, they no longer have to stay in abusive situations.

Disability Discrimination Act

The Disability Discrimination Act 1995 makes it illegal to discriminate against people on the grounds of their disabilities. The Disability Rights Commission gives information about rights in education, employment, and access to provision.

Research tip

In October 2007 the Disability Rights Commission, the Commission for Racial Equality and the Equal Opportunities Commission combined to form the Equality and Human Rights commission. Find out more at www.equalityhumanrights.com

Special Educational Needs and Disability Act 2001

Rights to an appropriate education and a statement of needs are set out in this Act and the Disability Rights Commission enforces this. The DRC provide information, help and advice to ensure those with special needs and disabilities are not abused.

Data Protection Act 1998

The Information Commissioner's Office is an independent body set up by the government to give help and advice to people about how to protect personal information.

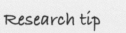

Research tip

Find out more about the Information Commissioner's Office: www.ico.gov.uk/

The Data Protection Act 1998 allows an individual to find out what information is held about them on a computer and in records. It gives the right to have the information corrected and also gives the individual a right to compensation if they are caused distress by incorrect information. The ICO helps people to exercise these rights.

Race Relations (Amendment) Act 2000

This amends the Race Relations Act 1976 to extend protection. Under the Race Relations Act, people have a right not to be discriminated against on the grounds of race, national or ethnic origin. The 2000 Amendment extended this to make public authorities promote race equality in services, and to improve equal opportunities in employment. The Commission for Racial Equality gives advice on these rights and minimises the risk of racial abuse by providing help and advice.

Care Homes for Older People: National Minimum Standards — Care Homes Regulations 2003

The standards are stated in section 23(1) of the Care Standards Act 2000. Standards 1-6 cover the choice of home; Standards 7-11 cover health and personal care; daily life and social activities (Standards 12–15); complaints and protection (Standards 16–18); environment (Standards 19–26); staffing (Standards 27–30); management and administration (Standards 31–38). This document makes it clear what older people are entitled to if they are in a care home or considering residential care. As these standards are set out in the Care Standards Act 2000, they are legally enforceable. Lay assessors as well as CSCI inspectors measure the quality of care by these standards. The potential for abuse is reduced when there are written guidelines to work to and when everyone has access to these standards.

POLICIES AND PROCEDURES

There are many working strategies to minimise abuse. We have seen legislation, policies and procedures aimed at minimising abuse. In this final section we will examine in more detail the POVA scheme we looked at above.

PROTECTION OF VULNERABLE ADULTS SCHEME (POVA) AND ASSOCIATED PRACTICAL GUIDE FOR PLACEMENT OF ADULT CARERS

The aim of the POVA scheme is to ensure that known abusers do not work in health and social care. The POVA scheme was originally implemented for:

- care workers employed by care homes, including agency staff employed in care positions where they have contact with care home residents

- care workers for domiciliary care agencies, who are employed in care positions concerned with the provision of personal care in their own homes for persons who cannot provide it for themselves without assistance.

Since 2004 the POVA scheme has been extended to cover adult placement carers. The POVA scheme set out in the Care Standards Act 2000 creates a list of people who are considered unsuitable to work with vulnerable adults in England and Wales. Care providers refer people to be included on the list and request checks against the POVA list as part of the application for a Criminal Records Bureau (CRB) disclosure for people they are about to appoint. Everyone applying to work as a carer in a home, as a domiciliary carer or for a care agency must be checked against the list before they start work. A care manager must get written confirmation that agency staff have been checked in the last 12 months. Checks are not transferable, so a carer must be checked every time they change employers.

Criminal Records Bureau and enhanced disclosure

Criminal Record Bureau (CRB) Disclosures are made under the Police Act 1997. There are two types of disclosure – standard and enhanced. A standard check gives information of criminal convictions, cautions, reprimands and warnings held on the Police National Computer. An enhanced disclosure gives this information plus any other relevant information held by local police authorities. Both types of disclosure can be linked to a POVA check. An enhanced CRB check is needed for those working in care, health and teaching.

Research tip

Find out more about the work of the Criminal Records Bureau from their website: www.crb.gov.uk/

If a CRB is applied for and that person is on the POVA list, the CRB inform the police and also tell the potential employer that they may not employ that person in a care position. It is a criminal offence to apply to work in care if on the POVA list.

Local and regional guidelines

Local and regional guidelines for staff and volunteers working with vulnerable adults are published by local councils.

Example

Birmingham local authority adult protection committee issued 'Multi-agency guidelines regarding the protection of vulnerable adults'. These guidelines work in conjunction with Birmingham Social Care and Health Directorate's adult protection procedures for the investigation of concerns that a vulnerable adult is being abused. The guidelines clearly state who does what and include a multi-agency referral form.

Research tip

You can see the multi-agency form and the guidelines on the Birmingham city website www.birmingham.gov.uk in the 'Adults and communities' section.

> **Think** What happens in your local area? Are there guidelines for staff and volunteers working with vulnerable adults?

Research tip

You can download both codes from the General Social Care Council website www.gscc.org.uk

The Nursing and Midwifery Council Code of Conduct is under review. Read the latest draft on www.nmc-uk.org/

Codes of Practice for Nursing and Social Work

In 2001 the General Social Care Council, the Northern Ireland Social Care Council, the Scottish Social Services Council, and the Care Council for Wales developed codes of practice for social care workers and employers.

The Code of Practice for Employers of Social Care Workers states the responsibilities of employers in regulating social care workers. Employers must meet the standards of their own code; support social care workers in meeting their code; take appropriate action when workers do not meet their codes. Employers have to maintain their own code and police the workers too.

The Code of Practice for Social Care Workers describes the standards of professional conduct and practice required of social care workers. Social care workers must protect the rights and promote the interests of service users and carers. This means treating each person as an individual; respecting and, where appropriate, promoting the individual views and wishes of both service users and carers. They must support service users' rights to control their lives and make informed choices about the services they receive. They must respect and maintain the dignity and privacy of service users, promoting equal opportunities for service users and carers and respecting diversity and different cultures and values.

The draft Code of Conduct sets out professional standards for nurses and midwives and outlines the duty of care they have. It states that they are personally accountable for their practice, for both actions – what they do – and for omissions – what they do not do. This means that a nurse who forgets to give a patient essential medication is breaking the code just as much as a nurse who accidentally gives too much. A nurse or midwife who breaks the code risks being struck off the register; this means they may not be allowed to work again as a nurse or midwife.

Here are some of the key points from the code:

Make the care of people your first concern, treating them as individuals and respecting their dignity:

- treat people as individuals
- respect people's confidentiality
- collaborate with those in your care
- ensure you gain informed consent
- maintain professional boundaries.

Work with others to protect and promote the health and wellbeing of those in your care, their families and carers, and the wider community:

- share information with your colleagues
- work effectively as part of a team
- delegate effectively
- manage risk.

Provide a high standard of practice and care at all times:

- keep your skills and knowledge up to date

- keep clear and accurate records.

Be open and honest, act with integrity and uphold the reputation of your profession:

- act with integrity

- deal with problems

- be impartial

- uphold the reputation of your profession.

> *Think* What similarities do you notice with the social care codes? What differences are there?

You may have noticed that nurses and midwives have professional accountability; they cannot say someone else told them to do something and so it is not their fault. They are accountable for their own actions or omissions.

EVIDENCE ACTIVITY

P5 – P6 – M3 – D2

For P5 you have to describe strategies and working practices used to minimise abuse.

For P6 you must identify the legislation, policies and procedures that protect adults receiving health and social care services.

For M3 you need to explain how legislation, policies and procedures contribute to the protection of vulnerable adults.

For D2 you have to analyse the role of multi-agency working in minimising the risks of abuse in health and social care contexts.

For P5, try to link the strategies and working practices to care contexts and give examples linked to case studies. There is a lot of overlap with P6 so try not to repeat yourself. M3 asks how, not what. Make sure you say how these all contribute to protecting vulnerable adults.

For D2, examine the role of multi-agency working in detail in terms of minimising risks to individuals and then analyse it. What are the strengths and what are the weaknesses? Link back to your placements. Was there evidence of joint working and joint planning? If so, did it work? How did they minimise the risk of abuse on your placement?

Public Health

unit 12

This unit is about public health, i.e. the health of the whole population rather than that of an individual. It is important for health and social care practitioners to understand how the health of the population can be protected and improved. They also need to understand the implications for their own practice and the impact on services and service users.

Public health covers a wide range of issues which affect the population. In this unit you will explore the history of the public health movement up to the present day. You will gain an understanding of the reasons for public health measures and examine current trends in ill health in the UK. The factors that influence health will be considered. In addition the key groups who influence public health and the methods of promoting, protecting and improving health will be explored. Examples of disease prevention and control are given as part of the unit but there are opportunities for you to undertake further research.

Learning outcomes

On completion of this unit you will be able to:

So, you want to be an...

Environmental Health Officer

My name Jo Fountain
Age 26
Income £27,000

If you want to have a direct impact on public health read on, this could be the job for you.

What do you do?

My training included food safety, such as ensuring that food is fit for human consumption, checking on food premises etc. I was involved in animal health which meant visiting pet shops, animal boarding kennels and the local zoo. Now I am specialising in housing. Also all the team undertakes educational activities – visiting schools, giving talks and mounting displays or exhibitions.

What responsibilities do you have?

I help to implement public health policies to improve the quality of life and promote a healthier society. I monitor the standards of public and environmental health and can enforce the regulations. At the moment I visit private and rented accommodation, including caravan sites, to see if the conditions are satisfactory. I sometimes need to take action to ensure improvements are made.

How did you get the job?

While I was at college doing A levels we had a speaker from the environmental health department talking about his job. I was very interested in his work and asked if I could do my work experience in his department. I applied to do a degree at university and was able to continue doing my practical experience locally.

> **"You have to be tactful and sensitive to the views of others"**

How did you find your current job?

When I qualified I was lucky to get a job where I had been working.

What training did you get?

During my degree I studied science, technology, statistics, social science and law at a general level. In addition we studied food, housing, environmental protection and public health in greater depth. I had to complete 48 weeks practical training which I did with my local department.

What are the hours like?

I work about 35 hours each week but the day is flexible. I sometimes need to work in the evenings or at weekends but I get time off in lieu.

What skills do you need?

Good communication and interpersonal skills are essential as you meet many different people. You have to be tactful and sensitive to the views of others. Other skills include the ability to make decisions and to be able to work independently as well as in a team, and a good standard of numeracy and IT skills.

What about the future?

There are so many options. But there are good career prospects to take up more senior roles. I could work in the private sector or for central government.

Grading criteria

The table shows what you need to do to gain a pass, merit or distinction in this part of the qualification. Make sure you refer back to it when you are completing work so you can judge whether you are meeting the criteria and what you need to do to fill in gaps in your knowledge or experience.

In this unit there are four evidence activities that give you an opportunity to demonstrate your achievement of the grading criteria

page 75   P1

page 83   P2

page 91   P3, P4, M1 and D1

page 99   P5, P6, M2, M3 and D2

To achieve a pass grade the evidence must show that the learner is able to...	To achieve a merit grade the evidence must show that, in addition to the pass criteria, the learner is able to...	To achieve a distinction grade the evidence must show that, in addition to the pass and merit criteria, the learner is able to...
P1 Describe key aspects of public health in the UK		
P2 Describe the origins of public health in the UK		
P3 Identify current patterns of ill health and inequality in the UK	**M1** Explain probable causes of the current patterns of ill health and inequality in the UK	**D1** Evaluate the role of factors that contribute to the current patterns of ill health and inequality in the UK
P4 Describe six factors that potentially affect health status in the UK		
P5 Describe methods of promoting and protecting public health	**M2** Explain methods of promoting and protecting public health	
P6 Identify appropriate methods of prevention/control for a named communicable disease and a named non-communicable disease.	**M3** Explain appropriate methods of prevention/control for a named communicable disease and a named non-communicable disease.	**D2** Evaluate the effectiveness of methods of promoting and protecting public health for the two named diseases.

12.1 *Understand public health strategies in the UK and their origins*

KEY ASPECTS OF PUBLIC HEALTH

Public health is concerned with the health of the community rather than the health of an individual. One of the key aspects of public health is to monitor the health of the population.

In order to do this it is necessary to understand the range of factors that can affect the community and its health. In 1991 Dahlgren and Whitehead used the following model.

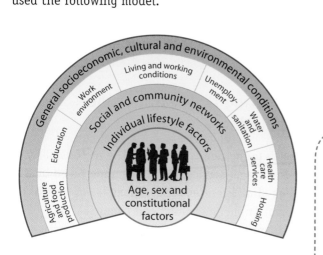

Figure 12.1 *Factors determining community health*
[Source: Dahlgren6. Whitehead M.1991]

Monitoring the health status of the community

Many different kinds of people are involved in public health. Local health services work in partnership with the local authorities and other agencies to monitor the health status of the community. Each region has a director of public health whose responsibilities include health improvement, health inequalities, health protection, health emergency planning, clinical quality and patient safety. Information is gathered from a number of different sources regarding the health of any population. Each year a profile of an area is produced.

Identifying the health needs of the population

Having assessed the health status of a community, it is possible to identify its needs. This may be done by making comparisons between similar groups. For example there may be a lack of services for one community compared with another. This is known as a comparative need. There may be the need to meet some external requirements or new standards. This is called a normative need.

Example

The North London borough of Islington has worse GSCE achievements and more violent crime than the national average. Air quality, numbers of road injuries and deaths are also worse than average for England and are even poor by London standards. More of Islington's older people are supported to live at home than the London average. Estimates suggest that more people smoke in Islington but that there are fewer obese adults. Life expectancy is lower than average, death rates from heart disease, cancers and strokes are high. Islington has a high number of alcohol related hospital stays and many people in drug misuse treatment services.

Source: community health profiles Islington

Think The example above is a summary of the health status of the London Borough of Islington for 2006. What are the health needs of the local community?

Developing programmes to reduce risk and screen for early disease

Public health seeks to respond to the identified health needs of a population by developing programmes that reduce risk. This may also include screening programmes to detect early signs of disease, which may be delivered by many different agencies or individuals. Examples might include:

- reducing the risks from drink driving by the police

- flu immunisation campaign by nurses

- physical exercise for children at school

- breast screening using mobile radiography unit.

Think Review the health risks identified for the borough of Islington. What sort of programmes might be developed?

Controlling communicable disease

Communicable diseases are caused by a micro-organism such as a virus or bacteria and can be transmitted from one person to another. There are different methods of transmission as a disease can be passed on:

- in droplets of water, saliva or mucus

- through food which has become contaminated

- through water which has become contaminated

- by direct contact including sexual contact

- by a vector such as a rat or mosquito.

Some airborne infections, such as the common cold, are not regarded as serious enough to warrant intervention. But diseases such as measles or tuberculosis have serious effects on individuals. Food poisoning occurs when bacteria such as Salmonella infect food; normally present in faeces, poor hygiene can allow it to be transmitted to foodstuffs with sometimes fatal results.

Contaminated water is responsible for high levels of disease. Public health interventions in the nineteenth century in the UK have ensured that the incidence of water-borne diseases is very rare. However, the United Nations reports that 4,000 children die every day as a result of diseases caused by drinking contaminated water.

Diseases that are transmitted by direct contact include fungal diseases such as athlete's foot. During unprotected sexual contact diseases such as HIV and syphilis may be contracted. Mosquitoes are an example of a vector that carries a disease from one person to another. Malaria is spread by this method as the mosquito transfers the protozoon Plasmodium between individuals. The WHO estimated in 2005 that more than one million people – mostly children – died from malaria.

Promoting the health of the population

Health promotion is not solely the responsibility of the health service but can be undertaken by a range of different agencies. Examples of health promotion include: childhood immunisation programmes; car safety schemes; healthy eating in schools and inspection of premises serving food. Tannahill (1990) suggested that health promotion had three aspects:

- health education, covering lifestyles, lifeskills and environmental education

- health protection, covering measures to ensure safety in housing, employment and food

- prevention, covering specific preventative activities such as screening and immunisation.

Individuals can be encouraged to improve their own health by making certain lifestyle choices such as taking exercise or not smoking. The role of public health in promoting health will be to influence behaviour and make social, environmental or economic changes which will lead to improved health.

Example

Lowtown is a deprived area with two secondary schools. A recent report has shown that the number of pregnancies and sexually transmitted diseases amongst teenagers in Lowtown has increased dramatically to well above the average for the rest of the area. Sally is a health promotion worker and has been asked to co-ordinate a plan to try to reduce the incidence. She has called a meeting to discuss how healthier lifestyles could be promoted among the young people.

> **Think** Who could be involved in promoting sexual health among these young people?

Planning and evaluating the national provision of health and social care

Public health is responsible for overseeing the quality of health and social care services. It does this by evaluating the services and ensuring that they are efficient and effective. It encourages a culture of evaluation of quality and of risk management. As part of the public health policy the government has introduced a number of standards for health and social care organisations, for example the National Service Frameworks (NSFs). These set the standards for certain groups and conditions and cover:

- mental health

- coronary heart disease

- diabetes

- older people

- children

- renal disease

- long-term conditions.

Organisations that monitor and regulate health and social care services seek to ensure the quality of services. For example the National Institute of Health and Clinical Excellence (NICE) and the Healthcare Commission.

> **Research tip**
>
> The Healthcare Commission provides an annual check on the quality of healthcare services. You can find out how your local services are rated by going to www.healthcarecommission.org.uk

EVIDENCE ACTIVITY

P1

For P1 you must describe the key aspects of public health in the UK. You will need to write an assignment that includes the evidence for P1.

Completing the following table will help you to structure your writing.

Aspect of public health	Description
Monitoring the health status of the community	
Identifying the health needs of the population	
Developing programmes to reduce risk and screen for early disease	
Controlling communicable disease	
Promoting the health of the population	
Planning and evaluating the national provision of health and social care	

SOURCES OF INFORMATION FOR DETERMINING PATTERNS OF HEALTH/ ILL HEALTH

World Health Organization statistics

The World Health Organization (WHO) is an agency of the United Nations. It is the co-ordinating authority on international public health. One of its core functions is to monitor and assess health trends through its own research programmes and through the collection and analysis of data from government sources. Examples of statistics produced by the WHO include:

- World health statistics, i.e. those related to the health of the 192 member states, such as demographic and socio-economic indicators; lifestyle and environment indicators; mortality, morbidity and disability; hospital discharges; and healthcare resources.

- Centralised information system for infectious diseases (CISID): information on communicable diseases, immunisation and recent outbreaks.

- Tobacco control database: information on smoking and non-smoking policies.

- Database of public health reports of member countries.

It is also responsible for providing an internationally accepted classification of diseases.

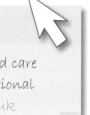

Research tip

You could look at some of the WHO statistics by going to www.who.int/whosis

Government statistics

The government collects a wide range of information about the population of the UK. The Office for National Statistics (ONS) measures the population of the UK and describes its composition.

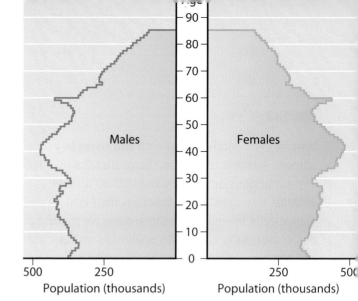

Population (thousands)   Population (thousands)

Figure 12.2 Population: by gender and age, mid-2005 Source: www.statistics.gov.uk

Research tip

Find out more about health and care reports from the Office for National Statistics www.statistics.gov.uk

Regional statistics

Statistics are also collected by region. The main regions in the UK are Scotland, Wales, Northern Ireland and in England the nine Government Office Regions (GOR): London, East, South East, South West, East Midlands, West Midlands, Yorkshire and Humber, North East and North West. Representing the national government departments they are involved in improving public health along with other issues such as fighting crime and supporting communities. The Regional Public Health Groups work with public health specialists in the NHS, local government and other agencies to address all the determinants of health. Regional Trends is a publication providing official statistics covering many aspects of life within each region.

Research tip

Regional Trends can be found on the website of the Office for National Statistics. Information about the English regional offices can be found at www.gos.gov.uk

Local statistics

Statistics are also collected by health and local authorities to meet the specific needs of a local population. For example in 2003-2005 Glasgow City had the lowest male life expectancy at 69.9 years while Kensington and Chelsea (in London) had the highest at 82.2 years. You will be able to find local statistics on the ONS website as well.

> ***Think*** The local registrar of birth, marriages and deaths collects data. Why might these statistics be useful in public health?

Epidemiological studies

Epidemiology is the study of the spread of disease and illness and the causes of death and disability in a population. It looks at patterns and trends of disease. Statistics that are used include:

- mortality rates (number of people who have died from a disease)

- morbidity rates (number of people who get a disease)

- incidence of a disease (number of new cases of a disease)

- prevalence of a disease (total number of cases of a disease)

- amount of disability in a community

- levels of well being.

They may also study lifestyle factors such as smoking and alcohol use or the economic, social and environmental factors affecting a population.

> ***Think*** Look at the graph showing patterns of death from 1911-2003. What reasons can you think of to explain the trends?

Regional reports

Each region produces reports on the population which they represent. These include information that is important for public health such as housing or transport. Annual reports, reviews and business plans are published.

Local reports

Reports about local public health issues are produced by a range of organisations. For example, local councils have responsibility for many services that affect the health of the local community. An example is the provision of recreational space. Reports are given at council meetings and are available to the public. Some issues will be reported in local newspapers.

Demographic data

Demography is the study of the growth, size, distribution, movement and composition of human populations. In order to understand the local community and its needs epidemiologists first need to know its basic characteristics, for example the size of its population and its age, ethnic and gender profile. One of the main sources of demographic data comes from the official census. This is a survey of the whole population which takes place once every ten years.

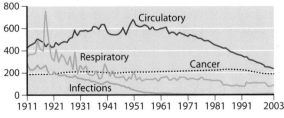

Rate per 100,000 population

Figure 12.3 Age-standardised mortality rates for selected broad disease groups, 1911-2003, England and Wales

Research tip

Visit the ONS website again to see what information was collected at the 2001 census which would be useful for public health.

Public Health Observatories

In 2000 the Department of Health set up nine Public Health Observatories based in each region and managed by the Regional Director of Public Health. Their role is to:

- monitor disease patterns and trends
- analyse data existing data to give early warning of emerging health problems and changes in health trends
- evaluate the impact of local actions in improving health and tackling health inequalities.

In addition to working for its own region each Public Health Observatory has a national role for specific aspects of health. Some have responsibility for linking with key national organisations.

Health Protection Agency

The Health Protection Agency (HPA) is an independent body that protects the health and well-being of the population. The Agency plays a critical role in protecting people from infectious diseases and in preventing harm when hazards involving chemicals, poisons or radiation occur. The agency also prepares strategies for new and emerging threats, such as a bio-terrorist attack or a virulent new strain of disease.

Research tip

Look at the website for the Health Protection Agency – www.hpa.org.uk

HISTORICAL PERSPECTIVES OF THE PUBLIC HEALTH SYSTEM

Public health has been a concern for communities throughout the history of the civilised world. In the UK the nineteenth century is seen as the 'golden age' of public health, when many institutions committed to improving public health were founded.

Public health in the nineteenth century

Two individuals are particularly remembered for their work in public health.

John Snow (1813–1858)

When John Snow qualified as a doctor it was assumed that cholera was spread through the air – the miasma or 'bad air' theory. He thought that it was a water-borne disease and in 1849 published a paper suggesting that cholera was a contagious disease passed on through the vomit and faeces of infected individuals. If the clean water supply is not kept separate from sewage widespread epidemics can occur. In 1854, when London was in the grip of a cholera epidemic, Snow was able to prove this in what has become known as the Broad Street pump theory.

Key words

contagious – a disease that can be caught from other people either through the air, from surfaces other people have touched, through food or contaminated water.

Snow thought that the cause of the cholera was probably the drinking water. He researched where people lived and identified which water pump was being used. By removing the handle from the pump he was able to demonstrate an immediate fall in the number of cases of cholera. This made health campaigners concentrate on improving the water and sewerage infrastructure.

Edwin Chadwick (1800–1890)

Edwin Chadwick was a civil servant during the Industrial Revolution in the UK, when many thousands of workers moved into towns to work in the factories. They often lived in cheap, crowded housing with little or no sanitation and disease was rife. In 1830 the average life expectancy for factory workers in Bolton was 17 years. In 1842 Chadwick's research proved that life expectancy was much lower in the towns than in the countryside and he campaigned for reforms to improve public health.

Sanitary movement

The 'sanitary movement' describes the actions that were taken in the nineteenth century to improve public health. The poor conditions in which many town dwellers lived led to very high mortality. In the 1830s half of all children who lived in Manchester died before the age of five. Overcrowding, malnutrition, ill health and bad working conditions led to high levels of disease which although affecting the poorest to the greatest degree also caused death throughout the community. The work of reformers such as Chadwick introduced sanitation systems such as clean water supplies, drainage and closed sewage systems.

Poor Law Act 1834

The poor were seen as the responsibility of their local parish and many places set up 'workhouses' where those who were unable to provide for themselves or their families were housed. In 1832 a Royal Commission was set up to review the conditions in which the poor lived. Edwin Chadwick was the assistant commissioner. Their findings resulted in the Poor Law Amendment Act of 1834 which aimed to improve the conditions of the poor.

> *Think* Why do you think the nineteenth century is known as the 'golden age' in public health?

The first Public Health Act 1848

The Public Health Act 1848 was passed to promote the health of the population and to improve sanitary conditions in the towns of England and Wales. It provided the basis for many subsequent developments in public health. It identified the major public health issues of the time, established structures that were to be responsible for ensuring improvements and set up national and local boards of health.

The local board of health was given responsibilities for sewers, street cleaning, public lavatories, slaughterhouses, street paving, public recreation spaces, water supplies and the burial of the dead.

Twentieth-century public health

During the twentieth century there was much greater emphasis on the biological causes of ill health and the social and environmental factors were seen as less important.

Beveridge Report 1942

The Beveridge Report is seen as the basis of the modern welfare state. It recommended a system of social security which would fight the five 'giant evils' of 'Want, Disease, Ignorance, Squalor and Idleness'. It was proposed that all working people should pay a national insurance contribution. In return those who were sick, unemployed, retired or widowed would be given benefits so that there would be a minimum standard of living for everybody. In addition a national health service would provide for the health needs of the population.

Key words

welfare state – a system of taxation which allows the government of a country to provide social services such as health care, unemployment pay, etc. to people who need them. Britain has a Welfare State.

National Health Service 1948

The National Health Service came into being in July 1948. It was to provide healthcare for all citizens, based on need – not the ability to pay. Before this, most doctors and hospitals charged for their services. Poor people often went without treatment because they could not afford to pay or relied on ineffective home remedies.

> *Think* What do you think is meant by the principle of 'free health care at the point of use'?

Acheson Report 1998

In 1998, fifty years after the founding of the NHS, Sir Donald Acheson published a report on the inequalities in health that still existed in society. He found that the health gap between rich and poor had widened. Coronary heart disease, stroke, lung cancer and suicide were higher for men in the lower social classes while for women the mortality gap was most marked for lung cancer and respiratory disease. The incidence of premature death, obesity, high blood pressure, accidents and mental health problems is higher among the poor and unskilled than among the well-off. In the early 1970s the mortality rate for unskilled men of working age was almost twice that for professional men. By 1998 it was almost three times higher.

Acheson found that inequalities in health were directly linked to inequalities in income. Children were disproportionately affected with one in three living in poverty. Often money allocated for food was used to meet emergencies, forcing mothers to sometimes go without eating. Families could not always get fresh food as supermarkets were built on out-of-town sites with poor transport links. Housing conditions in certain areas were poor and traffic pollution also caused ill health. The Acheson Report made it clear that health inequalities still existed despite the general improvement in life expectancy and national prosperity.

'Our Healthier Nation' (1999)

In 1999 the Labour government published a White Paper entitled 'Saving Lives – Our Healthier Nation'. It set out proposals for promoting healthier living, reducing health inequalities and saving lives. It set targets for 2010 in four main areas:

- cancer – to reduce the death rate in people under 75 by at least a fifth

- coronary heart disease and stroke – to reduce the death rate in people under 75 by at least two-fifths

- accidents – to reduce the death rate by at least a fifth and serious injury by at least a tenth

- mental illness – to reduce the death rate from suicide by at least a fifth.

Other areas to be tackled were sexual health, drugs, alcohol, food safety and communicable diseases. Actions were to include greater investment in health services, reduction of smoking in the population, integrating central and local government and including health improvement as a target for the NHS. It recognised that social, economic and environmental factors all affect health as well as the choices that an individual makes about their own health behaviours.

> **Think** How did the white paper 'Our Healthier Nation' provide a response to the Acheson Report?

Twenty-first century public health

In 2000 the government started a programme of huge investment in the NHS called the NHS Plan. Further White Papers and new organisations have been set up to address the issues of health.

'Choosing Health – making healthier choices easier' (2004)

The aim of this White Paper was to make it easier for people to choose to live healthy lives. The areas of smoking, obesity, exercise, alcohol consumption, sexual and mental health were identified as being the most important targets. The plans included providing information so that individuals can make their own informed choices. Poorer communities were to be particularly targeted. Sales of cigarettes, unhealthy foods and alcohol were to be restricted – especially to children and young people. Schools were encouraged to provide healthier foods, promote exercise and use school nurses to promote health. Workplaces were encouraged to help their employees to stay healthy.

> **Research tip**
>
> You can read more about 'Choosing Health – making healthier choices easier 'by going to www.dh.gov.uk

Public health agencies

Public health issues are not only the responsibility of local or national organisations. The consequences of pollution or the spread of infection can be felt world-wide. The World Health Organization was founded in 1948 and has a key role internationally in public health issues. The European Union is involved in public health issues that affect its members. National agencies that are responsible for aspects of public health include the National Health Service, government departments involved in housing, employment, education, the environment, agriculture, food as well as waste management etc. Local authorities also make decisions that affect public health. In addition some independent organisations lobby the government about issues of public health.

Health Protection Agency

The Health Protection Agency was established in 2003 to provide an integrated approach to protecting public health in the UK by giving support and advice. It seeks to protect the community against infectious diseases and other dangers to health such as chemicals, poisons or radiation. In addition it prepares for new or emerging threats such as a terrorist attack using biological weapons or a new strain of a disease.

National Institute of Health and Clinical Excellence

The National Institute of Health and Clinical Excellence (NICE) is an independent organisation which gives guidance on health and how to prevent or treat ill health. Its three main areas of work are public health, health technologies and clinical practice.

Research tip

In 2007 NICE is due to publish new public health guidance on promoting health and preventing illness. You can read about it at www.nice.org.uk

Target setting

Targets for improvement of public health are set at local, national and international levels. For example the local council or Primary Care Trust may set targets to increase participation in health-related activities such as exercise or to reduce the numbers of local people experiencing ill health. At national level the government has set a wide range of targets to improve the health of the nation and at international level the World Health Organization and the United Nations have set targets for their member states.

KEY GROUPS IN INFLUENCING PUBLIC HEALTH POLICY

Pressure groups

A pressure group is an independent organisation that campaigns on a particular issue or on behalf of a certain group of people. It aims to influence public policy and especially governmental legislation, regarding its particular concerns and priorities. Examples of such groups who are involved in public health issues are Greenpeace, Friends of the Earth and Oxfam.

Greenpeace

The Greenpeace mission statement is: 'Greenpeace stands for positive change through action. We defend the natural world and promote peace.'

Research tip

You can find out more about Greenpeace on their website www.greepeace.org.uk

Think In what ways does Greenpeace act as a pressure group for public health?

Friends of the Earth

Friends of the Earth wants the government to pursue policies that protect people and the planet. Their campaigns are on a local and regional level and include: working towards greener farming and a five-year ban on genetically modified (GM) food; campaigning for increased recycling and against more incinerators and landfill sites; working to reduce the impact on the environment of the movement of people and goods in the UK.

> **Research tip**
>
> You can find out more about Friends of the Earth from their website – www.foe.co.uk

International groups

International groups such as the World Health Organization and United Nations have a powerful role in public health.

World Health Organization

In its constitution the World Health Organization (WHO) sets out its objective as the attainment by all peoples of the highest possible level of health. Health is defined as a state of complete physical, mental and social well-being and not merely the absence of disease or infirmity. The WHO collects information about health trends and the causes of ill health and proposes actions to improve health across the world.

> **Example**
>
> The WHO's most recent 10-year plan is entitled 'Engaging for health.' It has the following seven areas for action:
>
> - investing in health to reduce poverty
> - building individual and global health security
> - promoting universal coverage, gender equality and health-related human rights
> - tackling the determinants of health
> - strengthening health systems and equitable access
> - harnessing knowledge, science and technology
> - strengthening governance, leadership and accountability.

> **Research tip**
>
> You can find out more about the World Health Organization from its website – www.who.int

United Nations

The United Nations (UN) is made up of 192 independent states. Its aims are to facilitate international co-operation in security, the rule of law, economic development, social progress and human rights. It seeks to prevent war, improve living standards, promote health and fight disease. The UN helps in the battle against AIDS, malaria, tuberculosis and infant and maternal mortality.

Example

Actions that the UN has taken which affect public health include the UN Conference on Environment and Development (the Earth Summit) in June 1992, which led to the creation of the UN Commission on Sustainable Development. It also declares and coordinates international remembrance days such as World Water Day, World Tuberculosis day, World Mental Health day and World AIDS Day. It provides humanitarian support through its World Food Programme which helps to feed more than 100 million people a year in 80 countries Work with refugees takes place in over 116 countries and peacekeeping is undertaken in over 24 countries.

Research tip

You can find out more about some of the organisations that make up the UN, such as UNESCO and UNICEF, by going to its website – www.un.org

National groups

In addition to the NHS, there are organisations in the UK with responsibilities for public health at a national level. They will influence the public health policies that are promoted by the national and local government. We have already looked at the Health Protection Agency and NICE. They are consulted and issue guidelines when government policies are developed. There are also agencies which look at specific diseases to try to find cures and better treatment. They can provide information that may influence policies on public health.

Cancer Research UK

Cancer Research UK is the world's largest independent organisation dedicated to cancer research. Its work includes researching how to prevent, diagnose and treat different kinds of cancer through the work of more than 3,000 scientists, doctors and nurses. Working in partnership with others, it seeks to have an impact both nationally and globally by campaigning and lobbying to keep cancer at the top of the health agenda and trying to influence government policy. It does this by providing expert evidence to Select Committees, groups of MPs and public inquiries. It also advises the Department of Health, NICE and other public bodies.

Research tip

Find out more about the work of Cancer Research UK at www.cancerresearchuk.org

EVIDENCE ACTIVITY

P2

Draw a time line to show the major developments in public health in the UK during the nineteenth, twentieth and twenty first centuries.

Describe how the need for public health strategies was recognized and how it has developed up until the present time.

12.2 Current patterns of ill health and factors affecting health in the UK

PATTERNS OF ILL HEALTH

It has already been suggested that patterns of ill health are spread unequally across the population. We will now look at some of the most important research that backs this up and the ways in which these inequalities are being addressed.

Black Report

In the 1970s the differences in mortality rates between the social classes began to be questioned. In 1977 a Research Working Group was set up, chaired by Sir Douglas Black, to look at both national and international evidence to assess whether inequalities in health existed in Britain. The review was completed in 1980. It concluded that at every stage in life the lower occupational groups had a worse experience of health. The Black Report suggested four ways in which its findings could be interpreted.

- The artefact explanation. The findings are not accurate but occur as a result of the way in which the data is collected. This is the explanation that the government of 1980 suggested was the reason for the differences between the social classes.

- Social selection. This suggests that those who are in good health get better jobs while those who are not so well remain in the lower social classes.

- Cultural explanations. Lifestyle choices and the culture of different social groups have an effect on the health and well being of individuals.

- Structural causes. Social structures affect the health of individuals. For example poor housing or poor educational opportunities affect health.

Black concluded that the last two explanations were the causes of the unequal patterns of ill health that were reported.

Example

Some of the findings about patterns of ill health that were published in the Black Report include:

- at birth and during the first month of life the risk of death in families of unskilled workers is double that of professional families

- boys in class V have a ten times greater chance of dying from fire, falls or drowning than those in class I

- mortality rates of males are higher at every age than females.

Think Why do you think ill health might be linked with social class?

Acheson Report

Published in 1998, the Acheson Report into health inequality mirrored the findings of the Black Report in finding a large gap in the health of the richest compared with the poorest in society. It concluded that one of the main causes of inequalities in health was poverty.

Examples of different patterns of ill health identified in the Acheson Report included the following:

- Over the last twenty years, death rates have fallen among both men and women and across all social groups. However, the difference in rates between those at the top and bottom of the social scale has widened.

- Infant mortality rates are lower among babies born to those of higher social classes. In 1994-96, nearly five out of every thousand babies born to parents in class I and II died in their first year. For those babies born in to families in classes IV and V, the infant mortality rate was more than seven per thousand babies.

- In the late 1970s, death rates were 53 per cent higher among men in classes IV and V compared with those in classes I and II. In the late 1980s, they were 68 per cent higher. Among women, the differential increased from 50 per cent to 55 per cent.

- Suicide is more common in men than in women, and in lower socio-economic groups. In 1996 the rates were three times higher for males than females.

> ### Research tip
>
> You can read more of the findings of the Acheson Report by following this link – www.archive.official-documents.co.uk/document/doh

Our Healthier Nation

On page 80 we looked at the targets set in the White Paper 'Saving Lives – Our Healthier Nation'. Examples of the inequalities that still exist included:

- Cancer – a third of all cancer deaths, and between 80 and 90 per cent of deaths from lung cancer, are caused by smoking. Forty per cent of unskilled men smoke compared with twelve per cent of men in professional jobs.

- Coronary heart disease – coronary heart disease is one of the biggest single causes of death with almost 115,000 deaths each year in England. The death rate from coronary heart disease in people under 65 is almost three times higher in Manchester than in Kingston and Richmond.

- Accidents – nearly one-third of deaths in 10 to 14 years olds are from accidental injury. Children up to the age of 15 years from unskilled families are 15 times more likely to die in a fire in the home than those from professional families.

- Mental health – suicide is the leading cause of death amongst men aged 15 – 24 years. Men in unskilled occupations are four times more likely to commit suicide than those in professional work.Governments have sought to tackle the inequalities in health experienced by the population in a number of ways. We will look at some of these.

A Programme for Action (2003)

This set out a plan to tackle health inequalities and their underlying causes. By targeting help to disadvantaged communities, the following were identified as likely to have the most impact long term in improving the health of the population:

- better support for families and children

- an improvement in educational attainment

- improvements to housing and help with heating

- easier access to public services

- reducing unemployment and improving the income of the poorest.

- reducing smoking and improving nutrition

- preventing teenage pregnancy

- managing the risks for coronary heart disease such as obesity, physical inactivity and high blood pressure

- reducing accidents on the road and in the home.

The plan was to improve the health of the poorest first but in addition raise the standards of health for the whole population. Although many targets were national, the Programme for Action expected local communities to work together to tackle the inequalities in their own areas.

> ### Research tip
>
> You can read more about the Programme for Action at www.dh.gov.uk

Choosing Health: Making healthy choices easier (2004)

Although individuals may wish to change their behaviour to a more healthy lifestyle, it is not always easy to do this. The government wanted to make it easier for people to make the healthy choice because it recognised that many inequalities in health are linked to choices that individuals make.

CASE STUDY: FAMILY DIFFERENCES

Alan and Mina met at university. Alan's family comes from a large manufacturing city in the north of England. He never knew his mother's parents as they both died before he was born. His grandfather died from lung cancer and his grandmother giving birth to her last child, his uncle. His father's parents are still alive. They live in a small bungalow and are reasonably fit, although his grandmother has severe arthritis in her knees – not helped by the fact that she is very overweight. Alan's Dad is about to retire from his job as a factory foreman. He smokes and takes little exercise. He has been told that his chest pains might be angina. Alan's mother has worked hard to care for him and his four brothers and sisters. She lost her job when the company in which she worked closed down and she was unable to get any other work. This has made her depressed at times. Money is often short and Alan tries not to ask them for any help.

Mina's parents are both doctors. Her home is in an affluent part of the south east of England. Both sets of grandparents are alive and very active. Mina's mother's parents both enjoy playing golf and take frequent holidays abroad. Her father's mother has arthritis but she has had a hip replacement and is fully involved in her active lifestyle, helping with various charities and doing her garden. Mina's other grandfather is about to retire after a successful business career in London. Mina has two brothers. When they were growing up they all enjoyed sport and horse riding. Her mother is a good cook and ensures that the family has a very well balanced diet.

QUESTION

How might inequalities in health affect Alan's and Mina's families?

FACTORS AFFECTING HEALTH

Research has identified that our health is affected by a number of different factors: socio-economic, environmental and genetic.

Socio-economic

You could refer back to Unit 7 to look at some of the social factors that influence health. They are shown in the spider diagram below.

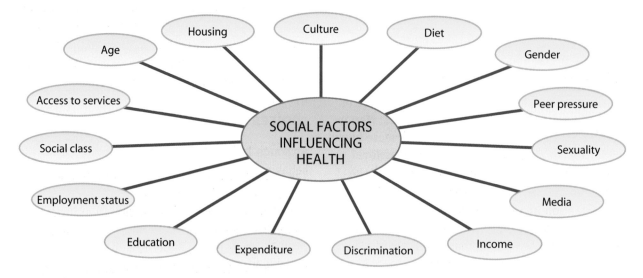

Figure 12.4 Health is affected by many different social factors

Social class

A person's social class means their social and economic level in society. Individuals and groups are classified by reference to their occupation. The Office for National Statistics uses a scale of eight different social classes. Previously the Registrar General's classification used five social classes. When checking statistics you may find that either is used depending when the research was undertaken. People who are in the same social class are likely to live in similar ways. Analysis has shown that they therefore experience similar patterns of health and illness. For example it has been shown that manual workers die younger.

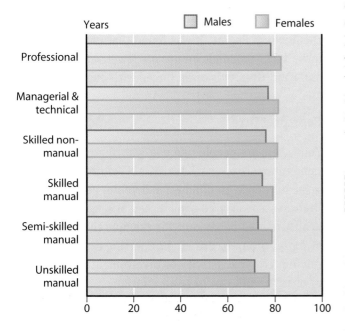

Figure 12.5 Life expectancy at birth, 1997–99
Source: www.statistics.gov.uk

Age

It is to be expected that as an individual ages they will experience more ill health but the patterns have changed significantly over the years. The average life expectancy in the UK has risen steadily. Better health care has meant that people can expect to live longer and in better health. Many infectious diseases which caused early death have been eradicated and so people may suffer from the diseases of older age groups such as cancers and heart disease. Advances in reproductive medicine have led to more premature babies surviving, but sometimes with complex medical needs.

Culture

Culture can influence customs, religion, values and norms, types of diet, social roles, knowledge and skills. Any of these can affect health. For example the type of diet someone eats or their attitudes to exercise may affect physical growth or rates of obesity.

Gender

Gender affects an individual's experience of health throughout their lives. Not only are there gender-specific diseases but men and women undertake different social roles in society, which bring associated health risks. Boys are more likely to experience accidents. By the age of 15 years boys have 65 per cent higher mortality than girls. For young male adults the rate is 2.8 times higher than for women aged 20-24 years. In adult life mortality rates are higher for men than women for all the major causes of death. Life expectancy for women is five years more than for men.

> ***Think*** Can you think why boys and young adult males have higher death rates than females?

Sexuality

Sexual activity and attitudes towards sex have an effect on the health of an individual. The rates of sexually transmitted diseases are increasing. There were 1.8 million attendances at genito-urinary clinics in the UK in 2005, twice that of the number in 2002. Reliable data on sexual orientation is not available though it is thought that about five per cent may belong to lesbian, gay or bisexual groups. Sex between men can be a major route for HIV infections.

Income and expenditure

The Black and Acheson Reports found that at every stage in life the poorest people in society experienced the worst health. The amount of money that an individual or family has affects their health and influences the choices that are made in how to spend it. The amount of money that is spent on food is disproportionably higher in poorer families, who may also have to spend a larger portion of their income on heating. Access to good food may depend on the use of a car and cheaper food may not be so nutritious. The use of leisure activities may depend on being able to afford entrance fees or the equipment required.

Employment status

The analysis of health inequalities and social class is closely linked to employment. Some occupations provide better opportunities and increase the health chances of individuals. Some individuals may experience short or long-term unemployment or may never work. These people experience significantly higher rates of long-term illness and disability. Later in life, retirement from work may affect people in different ways. For some it will be the opportunity to enjoy leisure while for others the loss of income and status may adversely affect their health.

CASE STUDY: EFFECTS OF REDUNDANCY

Bob had worked for the same firm since he left school. He had enjoyed his job and often met up with his workmates at the end of the day for a drink in the local pub. At the weekends he played football for the work team. Bob was very shocked when the company was sold and his entire department was made redundant. He has not been able to find another job locally. Many of his colleagues are talking about moving in order to find work. The football team has been disbanded and he does not feel like going to the pub as he no longer has a job. He and Sheila have few savings and he is becoming increasingly worried about the future.

QUESTIONS

1. In what ways might Bob's work have affected his health?

2. What changes might occur now that he has lost his job?

Housing

Housing was recognised as a factor in affecting people's health by Chadwick in the nineteenth century. In 1996, a review of houses in England concluded that 1.5 million homes were not fit for living in. The elderly, very young and those already affected by ill health are at risk. Unsuitable houses may be damp, have poor insulation and inadequate heating.

Diet

Good food is essential to health. Diet is a part of the lifestyle of an individual and the choices that are made may fundamentally affect their health and well-being. The effect of nutrition was explored in the Acheson Report. It was found that people in lower socio-economic groups ate fewer vegetables and fruit. Obesity is often linked with poor health.

Peer pressure

Your peers are people like you who share the same interests or characteristics. Peer groups have great influence on children and young people. Peer pressure may be good or bad and may affect health-related behaviour; for example the attitude of a peer group to drinking or getting drunk, driving, criminal activity or involvement in sport or charity work can have an effect.

Media

The media includes any printed or audio-visual material designed to communicate with others, such as newspapers, magazines, radio, television, billboards, exhibition displays, posters and leaflets. It can give information and raise awareness about health. It can have an immediate and powerful effect. Major health campaigns such as the winter flu immunisation scheme or road safety frequently use TV, radio and the newspapers top promote their message. The media also influences attitudes and behaviours. Issues about health can be raised indirectly, for example, through storylines in 'soaps' such as EastEnders. Celebrities may be used to endorse 'healthy' messages and firms may sponsor activities that are linked to good health such as sports events. Sometimes the media can have a negative effect on public health. Fashion models have been seen as promoting unhealthy ultra thin body images which can be copied by young girls.

> **Think** What do you think about ultra-thin fashion models? Can they be linked to anorexia in young girls?

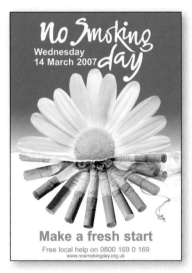

Figure 12.6 A media campaign that seeks to influence health

Discrimination

Unfair discrimination is when an individual or group of people receives less favourable treatment because of prejudice such as racism, sexism, homophobia, ageism or because of attitudes towards disability. It can mean that individuals do not get equal opportunities to access health services or receive the same treatment as others.

Education

Education can influence the health of individuals and communities. Health education is undertaken in many different ways and aspects of health form part of the school national curriculum.

Access to services

It is important that health services are accessible – not just in terms of location but also there should not be any physical or psychological barriers.

Environmental factors affecting health

One of our current big concerns is that of global warming. People are very concerned about its impact on the planet and particularly on the health of the world population. Worldwide, national and local environments all have an influence on their populations. For example there are differences between urban and rural environments. Water supplies and waste management as well as housing pollution affect communities and individuals. The provision and access to health services, as well as leisure and recreational facilities, can all affect health and well being.

Urban environments

An urban environment is one where a large number of people live, such as a town or city. During the nineteenth century many people moved into urban areas to get work in factories. Housing was dense and there was a lot of pollution. The health of urban populations can be affected because of over-crowding, pollution, higher crime rates, busy roads and more traffic. However, there may be positive effects on health with easier access to shops, health care and leisure facilities.

Rural environments

A rural environment means living in the countryside which is seen as less stressful with less air pollution. The smaller communities may mean that people know each other and can more readily give support. Negative effects on health may be associated with the lack of access to facilities such as health care or lack of transport.

> **Think** Do you live in an urban or rural environment? What are the possible positive and negative effects of living where you do?

Water supply

The work of public health reformers, such as Chadwick in the nineteenth century, ensured that water was made safe in the UK. We take for granted that our tap water will not cause illness. All households have regular supplies and we can be certain that we have sufficient for both drinking and for hygiene needs. However in the developing world the United Nations has reported that 4,000 children die every day as a result of diseases caused by drinking dirty water. Micro-organisms and chemicals can pollute water supplies and insects such as the malaria-carrying mosquito live near water.

Waste management

Every year in the UK 300 million tonnes of waste is produced; a quarter of this is rubbish from households and businesses. It is important for public health that waste is disposed of safely as rubbish can be a source of infection, contamination and other dangers. The management of waste is the responsibility of the government working through the Environment Agency and local authorities. It is policy to reduce waste and to recycle as much as possible. Households are asked to work with local waste management companies to reduce their own waste and to help with recycling such items as glass, cans, plastics and papers. There are strict laws about disposal of waste.

> *Think* What is done in your area to manage the waste from households?

Housing

The environmental impact of housing can affect health. Over crowding or buildings that are near to unsafe environments can affect people's health. Housing developments need to be carefully planned to ensure that the area can sustain the community and there will not be an over-demand on essential services. House building is strictly regulated through the local authority to ensure that buildings meet requirements for safety including fire safety.

Pollution

Air, water and noise pollution can all affect the health of a community. Air pollution is caused through emissions from cars, factories and households. The levels of air pollution have remained high in the UK and are thought to contribute to respiratory diseases, particularly asthma. Tobacco smoke used to be a major cause of air pollution but stricter rules have reduced the incidence and from July 2007 smoking will not be allowed in any enclosed public space. Water pollution occurs through the accidental or unregulated discharge of contaminates into the water supply. For example chemicals and pesticides can get into rivers and other water sources. Noise pollution applies to levels of noise that cause psychological or physical damage.

Access to health and social services

People can only receive good quality health care if they can access the services. This not only means where the services are situated geographically but also whether there are any barriers to access, such as transport difficulties, or physical barriers such as inadequate access for those with disabilities. Financial concerns may prevent individuals from using some services while others may find psychological barriers.

> *Think* Where are your local health and social care services based?

Access to leisure/recreational activities

Leisure and recreational activities can affect many aspects of health. For example, physical health can be improved through sport while social and emotional health can be supported through social interaction and friendships. However, people can only have access to such activities if they are available and affordable. Private health clubs can provide very good facilities but only for those who can afford to pay.

Genetic factors affecting health

Genetic or inherited factors can affect health. Some disorders are almost exclusively hereditary while others have both a hereditary and an environmental cause. This means that some people will be more likely to get certain diseases compared with others in the population. Medical research is discovering more examples of genetic links. For example, some forms of breast cancer have been shown to be inherited. If this is recognised early enough, preventative treatment can be given.

Sickle cell anaemia

This is an inherited disease. In those who are affected, the red blood cells, which are usually shaped like discs, become crescent or 'sickle' shaped. As a result they do not pass through the blood vessels smoothly but cause small blood clots. These are very painful. The disease is much more common in certain ethnic groups, such as those from African descent. The disease is present from birth although the symptoms may not occur immediately. It can be a life-threatening disease as the damaged blood cells break down, the patient becomes anaemic and there is damage to internal organs

Key words

anaemia – a medical condition in which there are not enough red blood cells in the blood

Thalassaemia

This is also a disorder of the red blood cells. People who are most likely to have the gene are those of Mediterranean descent, for example from Greece, Italy or Cyprus. It is an inherited disease in which the production of haemaglobin is insufficient leading to anaemia. There are two types – major and minor. The major form is very serious. Severe anaemia means that the patient has to have very frequent blood transfusions which carry their own risk.

Cystic fibrosis

Cystic fibrosis is an inherited condition. Some of the organs of the body, such as the lungs and digestive system, get clogged with sticky mucous. This makes it difficult to breathe and to digest food. In the UK over 7,500 people are affected. Cystic fibrosis is inherited when the child receives a cystic fibrosis gene from both mother and father. If only one gene is inherited then the individual becomes a carrier of the disease.

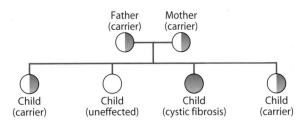

Figure 12.7 How cystic fibrosis is passed on

EVIDENCE ACTIVITY:

P3 – P4 – M1 – D1

For this assessment you need to look at current patterns of ill health and inequality in the UK and the factors that affect health.

In order to meet P3 you must identify current patterns of ill health and inequality in the UK. You will find information on the website for the Office for National Statistics. Identify at least 3 different patterns for example social class, ethnicity geographical area. You should use appropriate graphs that illustrate your findings.

For P4 you must describe six factors that potentially affect health status in the UK. You must cover examples from all three groups i.e. socio-economic, environmental and genetic.

For M1 you need to explain the probable causes of the patterns of ill health and inequality in the UK.

For D1 you must evaluate the role of the factors that contribute to the current patterns of ill health and inequality in the UK.

12.3 Methods of promoting and protecting public health

AIMS

Public health covers a wide range of issues that affect the health of the population. Overall its aims are to improve the health of the nation and to reduce inequalities. It does this through monitoring the health of the community and identifying its needs. From this analysis strategies are developed, which can be at international, national or local levels. The work tends to fall into three main categories:

- social – such as health promoting activities and health education

- protection – such as immunisation, screening for diseases

- environmental – such as waste management, water supply and pollution control.

HEALTH PROMOTING ACTIVITIES AND EDUCATION

Health promotion covers many different activities. It can be directed at one aspect of health or several. It may aim to prevent ill health, for example through discouraging people from starting to smoke. It may try to educate people about their current situation and what can be done, such as losing weight. It may try to help people deal with conditions that they cannot change, for example those with chronic conditions. The promotion may be directed at individuals to encourage them to improve their own health and that of their family. Public policies can be developed which focus on the health of a community or population. These may support individuals in making their own 'healthy choices'.

The aims of different programmes may differ. So the most appropriate methods will be chosen in order to meet the specific aim. The aims of health promotion have been categorised as follows:

- raising awareness

- providing information and improving knowledge

- empowering: improving self awareness, self esteem and decision making

- changing attitudes, behaviours and lifestyles of individuals

- societal change – changing the physical or social environment.

(Adapted from: Ewles and Simnet, 1992 Promoting Health A practical guide Scutari Press)

Example

Here are the ten tips for better health published in 'Saving Lives – Our Healthier Nation':

- Don't smoke

- Eat a balanced diet with plenty of fruit and vegetables

- Keep physically active

- Manage stress by, for example, thinking things through and making time to relax

- If you drink alcohol, do so in moderation

- Cover up in the sun, and protect children from sunburn

- Practise safer sex

- Take up cancer screening opportunities

- Be safe on the roads: follow the Highway Code

- Learn the First Aid ABC – airways, breathing, circulation.

Research tip

You can look at it in full 'Saving Lives – Our Healthier Nation' 1999 White Paper on www.official-documents.co.uk

There are many activities linked with health promotion and health education. Here we are going to look at two areas: healthy eating and the national No Smoking Day.

Healthy eating campaigns

Research shows that:

- obesity is responsible for more than 9,000 premature deaths per year in England

- obesity is a risk factor for diseases such as heart disease, stroke, some cancers and type 2 diabetes

- obesity in both adults and children is more common among lower social groups

- over half of all adults are either overweight or obese – almost 24 million adults

- obesity in children aged under 11 increased from 9.9 per cent in 1995 to 13.7 per cent in 2003.

Obesity is recognised as a serious problem for the health of the population in the UK. In 'Choosing Health – making healthy choices easier' the Department of Health set out plans to work with other government departments, the food industry and other organisations to raise awareness of the health risks of obesity and the steps that can be taken through diet and exercise to prevent it. The initiatives include:

- increasing the availability of healthier foods including reducing the levels of salt, added sugars and fat in prepared and processed food and drink

- increasing access to fruit and vegetables

- restricting the advertising and promotion to children of foods and drinks that are high in fat, salt and sugar

- ensuring that children in low income families obtain a healthy diet

- encouraging more women to breast feed as breast fed babies are less likely to be obese in childhood

- promoting local community programmes to increase physical activity.

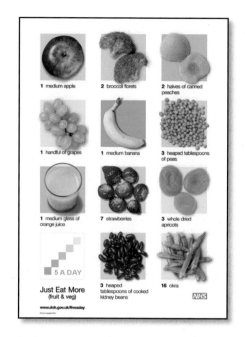

Figure 12.8 A healthy eating campaign launched in 2003

Commercial organisations may also promote their products as part of healthy eating campaigns. Food labelling allows individuals to make healthier choices by indicating the content of foods and the proportions of fat, salt and sugars. Other products are specfically developed to support healthy eating.

> **Think** In what ways is healthy eating promoted in your local shops?

Standards for school lunches

As part of the Five a Day programme a free piece of fruit was supplied for all four- to six- year-old children at school. In 2005 the government established the School Food Trust to work with schools and local authorities. Its remit is to transform school food and food skills, promote the education and health of children and young people and improve the quality of food in schools.

Research tip

You can find out more by going to the website www.schoolfoodtrust.org.uk

National No Smoking Day

No Smoking Day was started on Ash Wednesday in 1984 and has continued as an increasingly important national campaign. It is a registered charity and every year develops new slogans and images. Materials are made widely available to groups and organisations. Its vision is to reduce tobacco-related illness and death by supporting smokers who want to stop. This is done by providing an opportunity to stop and highlighting where they can get effective help.

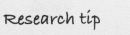

Research tip

More information and further examples of National No Smoking Day campaigns can be found on the website www.nosmokingday.org.uk

PROTECTION

The first measures that were undertaken by public health reformers were in order to protect the public from diseases. This still remains a key aspect of the work.

Immunisation programmes

Immunisation has eliminated many infectious diseases in the UK. However vigilance is still required to ensure that the uptake of vaccination programmes is sufficient to prevent an outbreak of the disease. Children are routinely immunised against a number of infectious diseases and people travelling abroad can obtain specific vaccinations to protect their health. Every autumn there is a campaign to provide immunisation against influenza in vulnerable groups such as the elderly.

The table below shows a timetable of vaccinations given to children in the UK.

Age	Disease vaccinated against
2 months	Diptheria, Tetanus, Pertussis (Whooping cough), Polio, Hib (a bacterium, which causes meningitis) PCV - Pneumococcal Conjugate Vaccine new from Sept 2006. Pneumococcal bacterium can cause pneumonia, septicaemia (blood poisoning) and meningitis, and is also one of the most common bacterial causes of ear infections.
3 and 4 months	Diptheria, Tetanus, Pertussis, Polio, Hib, Meningitis C
12 – 13 months	Hib, Meningitis C, PCV, MMR (Measles, Mumps and Rubella)
10 – 14 years	BCG against tuberculosis unless needed to be given earlier

Disease surveillance

The responsibility for monitoring diseases in the community rests with the Health Protection Agency Centre for Infections. As well as providing disease surveillance it coordinates the investigation into national and uncommon outbreaks of diseases. It provides advice about the risks from various infections and assesses the implications of any international health alerts. It reviews the success of immunisation and screening programmes. Its recommendations may lead to changes in public health policies.

The Agency receives reports from doctors and laboratories which are analysed and show the frequency (number of cases) and the distribution of any disease. Immediate action can be taken if necessary.

Example

Lyme disease is reported on by the Health Protection Agency. People can become infected after being bitten by hard-bodied ticks that are infected with a particular type of bacteria. Ticks become infected when they feed on birds or mammals that carry the bacterium in their blood. The HPA has given out information on Lyme disease so that people know how to protect themselves against it.

Research tip

You can find out more about Lyme disease on www.hpa.org.uk/infections/topics_az/zoonoses/lyme_borreliosis

Think How does this example illustrate disease surveillance and how the public's health is protected?

Screening

Screening is used to identify a disease early in its development in order to be able to provide more successful treatment or a cure. Screening starts at the beginning of a person's life with a number of tests during pregnancy to ensure the health and satisfactory development of the unborn baby. Other screening programmes check for early signs of cancer, for example cervical smears and breast screening. GPs have a regular routine of screening for high blood pressure.

CASE STUDY: BREAST CANCER SCREENING

Jill is 48 years old. She is due to start having routine mammograms to screen for breast cancer when she is 50. Both her grandmother and aunt died from breast cancer, while her mother was successfully treated for the disease. Jill heard that there are now tests to show if she has inherited a gene which would give her an increased risk of developing the disease. Her GP arranged for her to have the test. When the test came back as positive she was immediately sent for an early mammogram. This was clear but she will be regularly screened to make sure that if she does develop the disease she will be treated as soon as possible. Jill may also discuss with her doctor the option of having her breasts removed and having reconstructive surgery.

QUESTIONS

How has screening improved Jill's chances of remaining healthy?

ENVIRONMENTAL PROTECTION

This includes ensuring that waste is disposed of safely, the water supply is uncontaminated and that other forms of pollution are controlled.

Waste disposal and treatment

The amount of household waste has increased in the UK. The most common way of disposing of waste in the UK is landfill. Every year 111 million tonnes of waste goes into 4000 landfill sites. The waste decomposes and can release large quantities of methane gas. Some waste is incinerated but this can lead to potentially harmful greenhouse gases and other pollutants being released. However, some incineration plants can generate electricity from the waste. In response to the problem, waste recycling programmes have been introduced. The target is that the UK should recycle and compost

33% of household waste by 2015. There are strict rules regarding the disposal of waste that is regarded as hazardous.

Key words

hazardous – something that is dangerous and likely to cause damage

Supply of safe water

The Drinking Water Inspectorate is responsible for assessing the quality of drinking water in England and Wales. It can also take action if standards are not being met and the drinking water is unfit for human consumption. Water is supplied to households by different water companies but they are regulated by the Office of Water Services (OfWat).

Pollution control

The monitoring of the control of pollution is the responsibility of DEFRA – the Department for the Environment, Food and Rural Affairs. Regulations cover all types of industries to ensure that they do not cause pollution. Local authorities have statutory duties for local air quality management (LAQM) under the Environment Act 1995. They are required to carry out regular reviews and assessments of air quality in their area.

DISEASES

There are several different ways of classifying diseases but the way in which they are transmitted will affect how individuals can be protected. Communicable diseases are caused by micro-organisms such as viruses or bacteria. They are transmitted from one person to another. Non-communicable diseases are not passed on but may be caused by lifestyle factors, the environment or are degenerative diseases.

Key words

degenerative – an illness in which the body or a part of the body gradually stops working

Communicable diseases

All communicable diseases are passed on in the form of viruses, bacteria, fungi or protozoa. At some time everybody will have 'caught' a cold or flu. While most people recover quickly from the common cold other communicable diseases have much more serious effects and it is important to prevent their spread.

Tuberculosis

Tuberculosis (TB) is caused by the bacteria Mycobacterium tuberculosis. It can attack any part of the body but usually the lungs. It is spread through the air. When someone with TB coughs or sneezes the bacteria are out in the air and breathed in by others. People who have poor immune systems are more susceptible to the disease.

Improved living conditions first led to a reduction in the number of deaths from TB, followed by successful drugs to treat the disease. In the UK the BCG vaccination is successfully used to prevent the disease in most of the population.

Sexually transmitted diseases

The number of sexually transmitted infections has risen very dramatically in the UK. For example, between 1996 and 2005 cases of gonorrhea increased by 54% and chlamydia by 207%. Sexually transmitted diseases (STDs) are passed on during sex. There are at least 25 different diseases that fall into this category. The most common are:

- gonorrhoea
- chlamydia
- syphilis
- genital herpes
- genital warts
- HIV

The government set out a public health strategy for reducing the numbers of sexually transmitted diseases in 2001. Individuals are encouraged to practise 'safe sex', this includes the use of condoms and restricting the number of sexual partners.

Research tip

You can see an example of a campaign which aims to protect the sexual health of young people by visiting www.condomessentialwear.com

Meningitis

Meningitis is the inflammation of the lining around the brain and spinal cord. It can be caused by bacteria or viruses. Children and young adults are particularly at risk from the disease which in some forms can be fatal very quickly. Vaccines give protection against several but not all forms. As part of the childhood immunisation programme, children are vaccinated against meningitis caused by group C meningococcal disease, Hib, pneumococcal infections and meningitis caused by mumps and measles.

Salmonella food poisoning

Salmonella is a bacteria which is found in poultry, eggs, unprocessed milk and water. Salmonella food poisoning occurs when the bacteria present in faeces contaminates food eaten by someone else. This can happen if an individual fails to wash their hands properly after going to the toilet. It can cause stomach upsets with diarrhoea, stomach cramps, nausea and vomiting. Salmonella infections can be prevented by ensuring that all food is thoroughly cooked and that high standards of hygiene are maintained.

MRSA

MRSA stands for Methicillin-resistant Staphylococcus aureus. Staphylococcus aureus is a bacteria found on the skin or in the nose of healthy people. It is usually harmless although it may get into the body and cause boils or even blood poisoning. MRSA is a form which has become resistant to antibiotics. It is a particular problem in hospitals. In order to reduce the risk of spreading MRSA between patients the following routines should be followed:

- staff should thoroughly wash their hands before and after having any patient contact

- patients with MRSA should be kept away from other patients

- staff having contact with patients with MRSA should wear gloves and gowns which are discarded when leaving the room

- all areas should be regularly and thoroughly cleaned.

Poliomyelitis

Poliomyelitis is a highly infectious disease caused by a virus. It attacks the nervous system and can cause total paralysis very quickly. It mainly affects children. It enters the body through the mouth, multiplies in the intestines and is passed out of the body in the faeces. There is no cure for polio but it is prevented through immunisation. Since the polio vaccine was introduced in 1955 the number of reported cases has dropped steadily. The WHO has set a target of eliminating polio worldwide through a vaccination programme.

Measles

Measles is a very contagious disease caused by a virus. Complications can include severe infections of the brain and lung. It spreads through infected droplets being breathed in. There is no specific treatment for measles. However it is now preventable through immunisation and is included in the MMR vaccine. Unfortunately, more recently there have been some unsubstantiated statements regarding the safety of the vaccine. This has led to a reduction in the uptake of the vaccine and a corresponding rise in infections.

Non-communicable diseases

Many of these diseases can be avoided – or their impact reduced – by changes in lifestyle or an understanding of the way that they develop. Early detection can result in a cure or more effective treatment.

Skin cancer

Every year over 2,300 people die from skin cancer in the UK and there are 75,000 new cases diagnosed. There are two main types of skin cancer.

Malignant melanoma is the most serious type of skin cancer which develops in the outer layer of the skin. The first signs may be a change in a mole or blemish. If not seen early it can spread to other parts of the body and be fatal.

Most skin cancers are non melanoma and tend to affect older people. There are two types – basal and squamous cell. They are easily treated if seen early.

Research tip

You can find more about skin cancer and the Sun Smart campaign from the Cancer Research website
http://info.cancerresearchuk.org/
healthyliving/sunsmart

Lung cancer

Lung cancer is the second commonest cancer in the UK. It is almost exclusively linked with cigarette smoking, with nine out of ten people who are diagnosed with lung cancer having smoked. The most effective way to reduce the incidence of lung cancer is to stop smoking.

There have been many public health initiatives to reduce the numbers of smokers. They have included raising awareness of the dangers of smoking, restrictions on advertising, warnings on cigarette packets and laws enforcing no smoking areas.

Bowel cancer

Bowel cancer is the third most common cancer in the UK after breast and lung cancer. One risk factor is a strong family history of bowel cancer. Growths in the bowel called polyps can develop into cancer over a long period of time.

A national bowel screening programme is being phased in over 3 years from 2006. People between the ages of 60 and 69 will be offered the stool test every two years.

Coronary heart disease

Coronary heart disease (CHD) kills more than 110,000 people in England each year. Many of these deaths are preventable.

It is known that risk factors for coronary heart disease include smoking, poor nutrition, obesity, lack of physical activity and high blood pressure. All these need to be addressed in order to improve public health.

Research tip

Look at the 12 standards for CHD on the Department of Health website
www.dh.gov.uk

Stroke

Over 130,000 people in the UK have a stroke each year. Most are over 65 but it can happen to anyone. A stroke cuts off the blood supply to part of the brain, which causes damage to the brain cells and in turn affects different parts of the body and mind.

Strokes are most likely to happen to people who have medical conditions such as high blood pressure or diabetes but lifestyle factors such as diet, alcohol consumption, smoking and physical inactivity all contribute.

CASE STUDY: NO SMOKING?

Jade is 18 years old and studying at college on a health and care course. She has been smoking since she was 14. Her parents are both smokers and they only made half-hearted attempts to dissuade her from smoking. Recently her father has had a persistent cough and has been referred by his GP to the hospital to have a chest x-ray. They are worried that something serious might be found. This has made Jade review

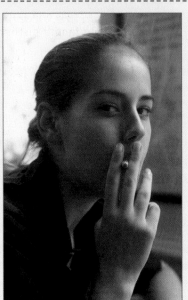

Figure 12.9 Jade

her smoking habits. She has learnt a lot about the effects of smoking on health as part of her course and become more aware of the warnings on her cigarette packets that say 'Smoking Kills'. Her college is a no-smoking environment and she often has to go outside in the cold and wet to have a cigarette. She works in a pub at the weekends and that is now banning smoking in order to comply with the law. As national No Smoking day is coming up Jade has contacted her local smoking cessation clinic to see if she could try to give up smoking from that day. Many of her friends are encouraging her and she hopes that she will find the willpower to stick to her resolutions.

QUESTION

1. What public health initiatives have been taken to reduce smoking?

2. In what ways have they helped Jade to plan to give up?

Diabetes

Diabetes is a condition when there is too much sugar in the blood. There are two types. Type 1 diabetes occurs when the body does not produce any insulin, necessary for the digestion of sugars into the body. This type usually occurs in children and younger people under the age of 40. It is not known why this type of diabetes develops. Type 2 diabetes occurs when the body still makes some insulin but not enough and usually develops in people over 40; it is associated with being overweight. Recently there have been more cases of younger people being diagnosed with Type 2 diabetes. Some ethnic groups such as African-Caribbean or South Asian people living in the UK are at greater risk.

Changes to lifestyle, such as improving the diet, taking exercise and losing weight may help to prevent the development of Type 2 diabetes.

EVIDENCE ACTIVITY

P5, P6, M2, M3 and D2

Using examples from each section – health promoting activities/health education, specific protection, environmental controls and protection from communicable and non communicable diseases, - describe the methods that can be used. (P5)

You need to explain how they work. (M2)

Choose one communicable and one non communicable disease to examine in detail.

For P6 you must identify the most appropriate methods of protection and or control for each of the diseases.

For M3 explain in detail the methods and for D2 you need to evaluate the effectiveness of the methods for promoting and protecting public health for each of the two diseases.

Working in the Social Care Sector

unit 17

This unit gives you the opportunity to explore social care careers, social care, organisation, administration and provision.

You will learn about the training, qualifications and personal attributes needed for careers in this area. The structure of social care services provision, and roles and responsibilities, including leadership and management, are explored. The policies driving holistic and integrated approaches to service delivery, multi-disciplinary working and regulations of the sector are examined.

When studying this unit you will benefit from work experience placements in the social care sector. This may be combined with the requirement for Unit 6: Personal and Professional Development in Health and Social Care, Unit 44: Vocational Experience for Health and Social Care, or Unit 45: Competence-based Vocational Experience for Health and Social Care.

This unit may not be combined in a programme with Unit 18: Working in the Health Sector

Learning outcomes

On completion of this unit you will be able to:

So, you want to be a...

Youth Worker

My name Hakan Callow
Age 26
Income £20,000

If you want to make a real difference to young people's lives then this challenging and rewarding job could be just right for you.

What do you do?

I work with young offenders under the age of 18. My job is to help prevent them from re-offending and to make sure custody is safe and secure. I help young people with issues such as health, education and employment and provide advice and guidance and sometimes referrals to more specialized help such as counselling. With some clients I act as a mentor and offer support on a one to one basis. I often work with a lot of other organisations such as the police, schools, and the Connexions service.

This is a job that can make a difference to a young person's life. It is varied and it is satisfying to see young people make the most of their abilities.

How did you become a Youth Worker?

You must be at least 18 years old to become a Youth Worker. I have a degree in youth work and community studies. As part of my study I completed field work placements which helped me to gain valuable practical experience. Occasionally people become youth workers without qualifications, and then train on the job. You will need at least one or two years of youth work experience usually in the form of voluntary work in the local community if you want to become a Youth Worker.

> **66 This job can make a difference to a young person's life 99**

What skills does a Youth Worker need?

You need a good understanding of young people and the main influences on their lives. You must be organised, with good communication skills, patience and a flexible approach. An ability to build a rapport with and provide support for young people is vital along with a strong sense of integrity and responsibility. Working with disaffected young people can be stressful so you need to be able to cope with that stress.

What are the hours like

I usually work around 37 hours a week; there is some weekend and evening work, probably about 4 to 5 times a year.

What's the pay like?

Newly-qualified youth workers earn between £15,000 and £18,000; more experienced staff between £20,000 and £25,000. Very senior staff can earn as much as £60,000.

What are your plans for the future?

At the moment I am happy where I am and I still have a lot to learn. In the future I would like to work as a youth worker with hard to reach groups such as the homeless.

Grading criteria

The table shows what you need to do to gain a pass, merit or distinction in this part of the qualification. Make sure you refer back to it when you are completing work so you can judge whether you are meeting the criteria and what you need to do to fill in gaps in your knowledge or experience.

In this unit there are six evidence activities that give you an opportunity to demonstrate your achievement of the grading criteria

page 110	P1, M1
page 117	P2
page 120	P3, M2
page 125	P4, M3
page 125	P5, D1
page 127	P6, M4, D2

To achieve a pass grade the evidence must show that the learner is able to...	To achieve a merit grade the evidence must show that, in addition to the pass criteria, the learner is able to...	To achieve a distinction grade the evidence must show that, in addition to the pass and merit criteria, the learner is able to...
P1 Describe the requirements for two careers in the social care sector	**M1** Explain how the requirements of social care workers can contribute to providing a positive experience for service users	**D1** Evaluate the requirements of social care workers in terms of providing a competent workforce in social care services
P2 Describe the overall structure of social care service provision in home country		
P3 Describe the roles and responsibilities of three overarching organisations in social care	**M2** Explain the roles of the three organisations in improving social care service provision	
P4 Describe three examples of legislation, policies, standards or codes of practice that influence social care service provision	**M3** Explain the role of legislation, policies, standards or codes of practice in improving social care service provision	
P5 Explain the role of workforce development in the social care sector		
P6 Describe two examples of multidisciplinary working in social care.	**M4** Explain how multi-disciplinary working can improve social care service provision.	**D2** Use examples to evaluate the effectiveness of multi-disciplinary working for service users.

17.1 *Understand potential careers in the social care sector*

The social care sector and the health sector are increasingly working together as care is integrated. When you study this unit you may find that the job of support worker is similar in each area. Care planning is very similar in both areas and so are management skills. There are some careers which are still specific to social care and we examine them here.

POTENTIAL CAREERS

Social workers are professionally qualified staff who work with individuals to assess their care needs and plan how to meet those needs. They monitor the care plan to make sure the care happens. Social workers generally have an honours degree in social work and register with the General Social Care Council. Social workers tend to specialise in either adult or children's services.

Social workers in adult services work with people with mental health problems or learning difficulties in residential care; work with offenders, supervising them in the community and supporting them to find work. They assist people with HIV/AIDs and work with older people at home to sort out problems with their health, housing or benefits.

Figure 17.1 Social workers work with a variety of people

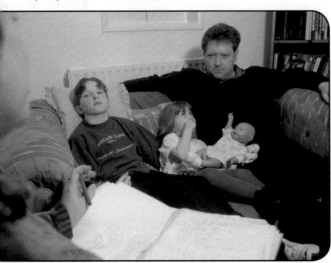

Social workers in children and young people's services give help and advice to keep families together; work in children's homes; manage adoption and foster care processes; provide support to younger people leaving care or who are at risk or in trouble with the law; or can help children with school or family problems.

Social care workers offer more personal care. They carry out the care that a social worker has planned. They may not need qualifications to start work but they will be expected to work towards a qualification such as a National Vocational Qualification as they work. Their employers will organise an induction and further training.

Care managers are usually qualified social workers or nurses. Sometimes a care manager of a residential home may have a Registered Manager's award at level 4. The job role of a manager in care varies. Sometimes a care manager manages a caseload of clients. In other care manager roles, they may manage a care home. Increasingly, care managers are professionally qualified social workers or nurses.

Support workers perform a variety of roles. They may work in the community supporting the work of the social worker. Sometimes they may help people with housing issues, or claim benefits to support them in living independently. Sometimes support workers work in hostels or supported housing. A Senior Waking Night Support Worker may supervise a small team, enabling tenants to gain the skills needed to move on into independent living. Part of the role may be to ensure the safety and maintenance of the building, observing and ensuring health and safety procedures.

Research tip

To find out more about jobs in the social care sector go to
www.socialcarecareers.co.uk
www.publicsectorcareers.org/

REQUIREMENTS: EDUCATION AND TRAINING

Education and training are needed for all social care work. The competence route involves on-the-job training such as National Vocational Qualifications. NVQs in health and care start at level 2 for care workers. Supervisors may need NVQ level 3. Care managers need NVQ level 4 care management. NVQs demand a blend of knowledge and skills which are assessed on the job.

> **Key words**
> --
> Competence – the ability to do something

The apprenticeship framework

'Young Apprenticeship pre-16' is a new route at Key Stage 4 which allows pupils to study for vocational qualifications in the classroom, in college, with training providers and in the workplace. The first Young Apprenticeship Cohort 4 Programme is in September 2007.

Apprenticeships consist of on-the-job learning plus education. Level 2 and level 3 apprenticeships include NVQ, key skills and an element of theory. Apprentices learn while they work, and train on the job. They attend college usually one day each week.

NVQs

National vocational qualifications are competence based. This means learners are assessed against a national set of standards. They are assessed on what they can do and either meet the standard or do not yet meet it. They can have another chance if they are not yet at the standard. People who are good at doing things rather than writing them down sometimes find NVQs suit them better. There are no age limits but carers must be 18 years old to perform personal care such as bathing people or helping them with toilet needs. NVQs are not fixed over a set period of time. Students can work at their own pace. An average time for an NVQ at level 3 may be 18 months but this can vary with individual students.

Work experience is essential for anyone taking an NVQ as they are assessed on what they can do in the workplace. An assessor observes the candidate doing their work and may ask the candidate why they did something. The candidate needs to know why something is good practice as well as what is good practice. If the candidate meets the requirements they are said to be competent. The role of the assessor is important in guiding and supporting the candidate at first so the candidate gets a clear idea of what they can do and what they need to improve on. The assessor helps the candidate to plan for assessment at a specific time then becomes the judge of whether that candidate is competent.

There are different levels of NVQs. Level 1 requires an ability to perform routine activities. There is no level 1 in Care because people are unpredictable. A person who is happy one day may be aggressive or violent the next and the worker must learn to cope with a variety of situations.

Level 2 requires workers to work under the direction of others. Level 3 requires workers to take more responsibility, supervising others. Carers who achieve level 3 NVQ may apply to university to do a nursing course. Level 4 is a managerial role requiring even more responsibility. Level 5 involves strategic planning and overall responsibility for an organisation.

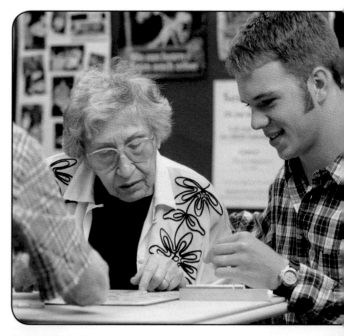

Figure 17.2 Apprenticeship allows young students to train on the job

BTECs

BTECs are work-related qualifications which were originally developed by the Business & Technology Education Council (BTEC), which became part of Edexcel. BTECs are offered as full-time courses from one to two years and also as short courses. BTEC qualifications are recognised and available in over 50 countries.

Level 1 –BTEC Introductory

Level 1 qualifications offer a broad introduction to a sector. They also provide a flavour of how BTECs work. An Introductory Certificate has four units: two core units, which everyone takes, a compulsory Personal Skills unit and one optional unit. The optional unit enables you to study an area in more depth. An Introductory Diploma has eight units: three core units, which everyone takes, two compulsory Personal Skills units and three optional units. The course usually lasts for one year.

Level 2 –BTEC First

Level 2 qualifications are good for those who have some GCSEs, but who want to do something different. They also develop skills and knowledge from Level 1. There is a certificate of three units – two core units, which everyone takes, and a choice of one specialist unit. The BTEC First certificate is equivalent to two GCSEs grades A* to C. The BTEC First Diploma is equivalent to four GCSEs grades A* to C. The Diploma is normally taken as a full-time course over one year. It contains six units – two core units that everyone takes – and four specialist units.

Level 3 –BTEC National

These qualifications are at the same level as A levels but can get you a job as well as a university place. BTEC Nationals are well known and recognised by universities. They carry UCAS points. A BTEC National Diploma is based on national occupational standards and usually takes two years. Eighteen units are studied and there are three mandatory work placements. It is also possible to take a level 3 BTEC National Certificate with twelve units, and a BTEC National Award with six units. The BTEC National Award in Health and Social Care is planned as an additional qualification within a level 3 programme with GCEs.

The BTEC National Diploma (from September 2007) has the following pathways:

- Children's Care, Learning and Development

- Health and Social Care

- Health and Social Care (Health Sciences)

- Health and Social Care (Health Studies)

- Health and Social Care (Social Care).

The Social Care pathway provides the opportunity for more care-based units for those students wishing to enter social work careers. The health and social care pathway offers a balance of units for those students who have not yet decided on a final career choice in health and social care.

Level 4 – BTEC Higher National/BTEC Foundation Degree

These are BTEC's undergraduate qualifications, roughly equivalent to the first half of a degree. A BTEC HND can get you onto the third year of many degree programmes but not into nursing or social work. Foundation degrees are planned for some professions allied to medicine.

Level 5 – BTEC Diploma in Management Studies

Level 5 qualifications are usually most suitable for managers wanting to gain more skills in a particular area. For example, the Diploma in Management Studies can take students onto an MBA course at Heriot-Watt University.

A-Levels, GCE in Health & Social Care

A-levels give a broad understanding of the sector, some skills as well as technical knowledge and an awareness of particular groups and their needs by focusing on Health, Early Years (Care and Education), Care of Older People, or Individuals with Specific Needs. Unlike BTECs, these qualifications have some examined units. They do not have the workplace element so students take a theoretical approach to many subjects.

You can study for a:

- Single Award AS GCE (3units): Units 1, 2, 3

- Double Award AS GCE (6 units): Units 1 to 6

- Single Award Advanced GCE (6 units): Units 1, 2, 3, 7, 8, 9

- Double Award Advanced GCE (12 units): all units.

Specialised diploma

The specialised diploma has been developed for 14 to 19 year olds to provide a more vocational approach to learning than the A-level route. The specialist diploma Society, Health and Development covers the area of Care. There are three parts to the diploma – vocational or principal learning related to care; generic learning which includes English and Maths as well as personal skills, and finally additional or specialist learning. The course includes practical activities such as visits, and a project which is internally assessed. The course includes ten days of work experience.

Levels of diplomas

The Diploma is available at levels 1, 2 and 3.

- Level 1 Diploma will be comparable, in terms of average length of study, to a programme of four to five GCSEs

- Level 2 Diploma will be comparable, in terms of average length of study, to a programme of five to six GCSEs

- Level 3 Diploma will be comparable, in terms of average length of study, to a programme of three GCE A levels.

- A level 3 award is also being developed, to be broadly comparable in size to two A levels.

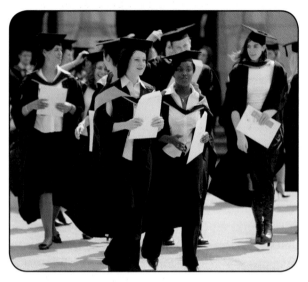

Figure 17.3 Social work now requires a relevant degree

Degrees

Degrees represent higher level study at level 4 or 5. Universities offer degrees on a full or part-time basis. Social work now requires a relevant degree and professional registration. It is possible to take a degree in social policy but not be a social worker and many people do take such a degree out of general interest. Sometimes a relevant degree may help to fast track towards a professional degree if a person later decides they wish to become a social work professional.

The best way to find out what degrees are offered is to check the UCAS website and search for the degree you are interested in. You can search alphabetically by course; for example, searching for Social Work brings up a list of universities which offer this degree. The University of York offers Social Work as a three-year full-time honours degree. This site also gives information about entry requirements, how to apply, and funding arrangements.

Research tip

You can find out more about UCAS by going to their website www.ucas.com.

Registration

The social care register is a list of those who are trained and fit to work in care. Currently social workers and students and eventually all social care workers will be on the register. Employers must check that anyone to whom they offer employment is on the register, and anyone using the services may also check that their carer is registered. The General Social Care Council regulates social care workers.

Knowledge sets

Knowledge sets are key learning outcomes for specific areas of work in adult social care. They were developed by Skills for Care, the workforce development body for adult social care in England in order to standardise learning for the adult social care workforce. They can be used by employers and awarding bodies to produce training packages that provide a standardised body of knowledge on a subject. They can be used with the Common Induction Standards (CIS) as part of continuing professional development and cover dementia, medication, infection prevention and control, workers not directly delivering care, nutrition and well-being, and safeguarding vulnerable adults. Progress logs are available to track progress.

Integrated Qualification Framework for the Children's Workforce

The Children's Workforce Network is a partnership of sector skills councils including Health; Education; Care; Sport and recreation; and Justice. It is led by the Children's Workforce Development Council. The Integrated Qualification Framework (IQF) must be in place by 2010 and cover most of the occupational roles in the children's workforce. It links to the Children's Workforce Strategy and the reform programme set out in *Every Child Matters*. The IQF will clarify qualifications and progression routes, encourage a better qualified and more flexible workforce and facilitate partnership working, in developing and delivering integrated services to children, young people and their families and carers.

> **Research tip**
>
> Go to www.childrensworkforce.org.uk to find out more about The Children's Workforce Network.

PRACTICAL SKILLS, KNOWLEDGE AND UNDERSTANDING

Much of this section is covered in detail in the core units:

- Unit 1: Developing Effective Communication in Health and Social Care

- Unit 2: Equality, Diversity and Rights in Health and Social Care,

- Unit 3: Health, Safety and Security in Health and Social Care;

- Unit 5: Fundamentals of Anatomy and Physiology for Health and Social Care

- Unit 6 Personal and Professional Development in Health and Social Care

Practical skills are what you do. Knowledge is what you know. Understanding is about knowing why. Take a simple example – you may be able to make a sandwich. That is a skill. Young children can learn to make a sandwich. Knowing what food groups are will help you to select healthy ingredients, so you may choose wholemeal bread and a salad filling for vitamins and fibre. Understanding why you need vitamins and fibre means you really are competent in delivering a healthy diet.

Care is a practical subject but skills alone are not enough. We also need knowledge and understanding. Communication is a skill requiring verbal and non-verbal abilities. Knowing what type of communication to use with someone who is visually impaired is important. Understanding why you must adapt your techniques is also necessary. A person-centred approach to care contrasts with an institutional approach and puts the client at the heart of the process.

CASE STUDY: RESIDENTIAL CARE

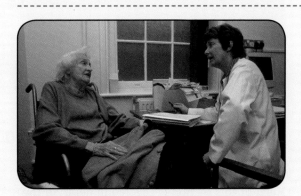

A client in a residential home became confused and aggressive. The carers thought she was just getting old, but as her behaviour got worse they became more concerned and they called an ambulance. The client was taken to hospital.

The nurse admitting the client noticed that her cheeks were bright red, and her lips were dry and cracked. The client's temperature was recorded as 38 degrees centigrade. The nurse managed to get a sample of the client's urine. It was dark, cloudy and smelled 'fishy'. The doctor prescribed antibiotics and plenty of fluids. Two days later, the client was lucid, pleasant and no longer confused.

If the carers had been aware that dry cracked lips and dark urine indicate a person has not drunk enough fluid, they could have given her extra drinks. If they had known that bright red cheeks may indicate a high temperature, they could have called the local GP and saved a hospital admission. If they had known that urine infections may cause confusion in older people, they may not have written off the client as 'just getting old'.

QUESTIONS

1. How could this situation have been prevented?

2. What policies should the care home adopt to ensure this doesn't happen again?

Basic anatomy/physiology should be understood by all who work in care. The case study above may help you to understand why.

Dietary understanding – knowing why people of different ages need different amounts of each food group – is vital if children are to get the amount of calcium they need for strong bones and teeth. This understanding is equally important in knowing how much food an older person who is inactive needs, and how much fluid they need. Coffee and tea dehydrate (take fluid out of the body). An older person who sits in a heated room all day is likely to need water to stay healthy.

Safe food preparation is essential when working with the young and old alike. Poor food hygiene can lead to sickness and even death in vulnerable groups. The responsibility for health and safety is everyone's, not just the manager's responsibility. Everyone must be trained but they must work safely, according to the procedures set out for their organisation. The employer has a duty to protect staff and keep them informed about health and safety. Staff have a responsibility to look after themselves and others. Health and safety is about preventing people from being harmed by work or becoming ill through work. Health and safety law applies to all businesses and covers employees, full - or part-time, temporary or permanent ; the self-employed; young people doing work experience; apprentices; charity workers; mobile workers and home workers including childminders. Moving and handling is part of health and safety.

Procedures for first aid will vary between organisations, but any employer with a workforce of 50 or more employees or in a high risk area must have suitable qualified staff who have a current first aid at work certificate.

By law, no one under the age of 18 years is allowed to assist with personal care such as a client's personal hygiene requirements. This is to protect staff and clients. A young person may not know how to manage the situation and may not be able to offer the best care to the client.

The use of aids and adaptations may vary from client to client and from organisation to organisation. A client at home may manage with a walking frame. A client in a care home may need a wheelchair. All clients have individual needs, which is why person-centred care is important. The carer must learn what is applicable to their area of work.

Duty of care

'Duty of care' is a legal obligation that requires each individual to exercise a reasonable standard of care when doing anything which could harm others. A carer bathing a client must check the water temperature before the client gets in the bath because water which is too hot may scald the client. When serving food, a carer has a duty of care to make sure the client is not allergic to the food. Some professions, such as doctors, judge any breach of a duty of care by a panel of other professionals, so a panel of doctors will judge a doctor accused of being negligent.

Procedures

Recording and reporting procedures form part of the duty of care. If a child is withdrawn and not eating, it is the duty of the childcare worker to record this and report concerns to the relevant people. The relevant person may be their line manager or sometimes it may be the parent. Procedures for sharing information vary depending on the care situation. Wherever you work, it is your duty to make sure you know the procedure in that situation. Parents of a child who has been taken into care may not be the first people to contact if a child is ill at nursery. Care planning processes should state the procedure for recording, reporting and sharing information. There are usually procedures in place which set out what to do and you should be told these during your induction. Care planning processes vary slightly between organisations, but overall there is a move towards joint working and sharing information where appropriate.

There is a common core of skills and knowledge for the children's workforce which is being set out in the Integrated Qualification Framework.

SOCIAL SERVICES – CARE PLAN
Date 23rd November 2007

Name – Claire Miller

We have agreed that the following services will be supplied to you	Supplied by	Monitored by
1. Accommodation	Utopia Housing Association	Social worker
2. Health – an appointment with the practice nurse for contraceptive advice	GP	GP
3. Social – opportunity to meet new friends at Rightside Youth club	Youth worker	Social worker
4. Education and training – Attend college for basic skills English and Maths	Utopia College	Social worker
5. Finance – help to apply for housing benefit	Youth worker	Social worker
6. Occupation – careers advice	Connexions Service	Social worker

Date for review: 4th January 2008

I agree that these services should be provided.

Signed by client............

Signed by care manager/social worker

Authorised by SSD..................

Figure 17.4 A care plan

Personal attributes

These are your personal qualities. There are some personal attributes that are essential for anyone who wishes to work in care. If you do not have these attributes already, you may need to work on them, and can plan how you will do this in unit 6 as part of your personal and professional development.

The ability to gain knowledge and skills is very important in care because care changes. A client may develop new needs. You have to be able to learn new ways of working to be a good carer. Joint working is a recent development in care. You will need good interpersonal skills to work with others and share relevant information. You have to use your initiative at times when people do something you did not anticipate. A child might throw a toy at another child. An older person may fall and injure themselves. You may be the nearest person and have to use your initiative to sort out the problem until help arrives.

Confidence is important. A child needs to know the adult is calm and in control. As a carer you may be faced with a situation where you feel uncertain, but you have to appear confident and in control so that you can calm others. A child who has just cut their knee does not want a carer who bursts into tears or panics. An older person who has fallen does not want a carer to stand and cry. They need practical help, possibly even an ambulance.

Empathy with others demands that a carer can put themselves in the client's place and know what they feel and need. Empathy is not sympathy.

Key words

Empathy is the ability to identify with and understand another person's feelings or difficulties

Think Just imagine if you had fallen and broken your wrist. Which would you rather have – a carer who stands and cries or one who gets help?

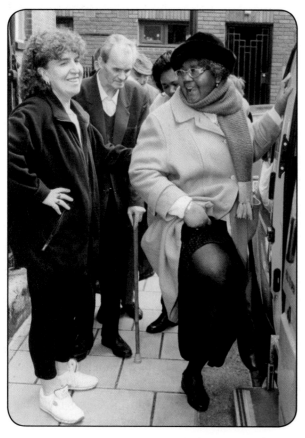

Figure 17.6 *The ability to work with others is one attribute a careworker needs*

The ability to develop an anti-discriminatory approach is a key attribute in care work. We cannot judge others and we cannot discriminate in care work. You may be called upon to care for someone who has hurt a child or hurt others. As a care worker you cannot say that you will only care for certain people. You must care for all. This is a core value. Some people find this hard to accept and for this reason may not be able to work in care.

The ability to work with others and to be reliable are two personal attributes needed for team work. The ability to take responsibility for oneself and for others are attributes needed to work in care. A person who cannot take responsibility for themselves cannot help others. Someone who always arrives at work late and blames others will not make a good care worker. Others cannot rely on them to be on time, or to work as part of a team without causing friction. In Unit 6 you will have made SMART action plans for your personal development. Perhaps some of these personal attributes may have been the focus for your plans. If you really want to work in care, you have to develop personally as well as professionally.

EVIDENCE ACTIVITY

P1, M1

P1 Describe the requirements for two careers in the social care sector.

M1 Explain how the requirements of social care workers can contribute to providing a positive experience for service users.

You are thinking of working in the social care sector but are unsure what career to choose so decide to look at two careers to help you make up your mind. You need to explain to parents how these requirements can help people. Write a brief report summarising your findings.

17.2 *Understand how organisations are structured in the social care sector*

The social care sector can appear confusing as there are many different organisations offering different types of care.

The Department of Health sets national standards and shapes NHS and social care services, promoting healthier living in England. Health and social care services are delivered through the NHS, local authorities, arm's length bodies and other public and private sector organisations. The Department of Health is accountable to the public and the government for the overall performance of the NHS, personal social services and the work of the Department itself.

KEY ELEMENTS OF HEALTH AND SOCIAL CARE PROVISION

The key elements of health and social care provision can be seen in the diagram below.

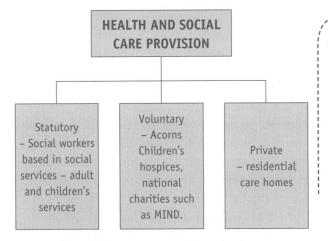

Figure 17.6 Organisation of health and social care provision

Statutory

Until 1990 most health and social care was provided by the state, i.e. it was statutory provision. Statutory, voluntary, private and informal providers of care became more equal partners in health and social care provision after the NHS and Community Care Act 1990.

Key words

Statutory means required by statute or written law; a state requirement

Statutory provision for social care in a community would include a local council social services department and a social services-run day centre.

Voluntary

Voluntary provision includes national and local charities. National charities such as MIND provide advice and support for people with mental health issues in England and Wales. A local charity may fund a hospice in a local area for those with a terminal illness.

Research tip

Find out more about the work of MIND by going to their website www.mind.org.uk.

Example

Acorns children's hospices are local charities which offer care in the West Midlands to life-limited children and their families 24 hours a day, seven days a week.

Acorns get over 80% of its income directly from the public. Less than 20% of their funding comes from government sources.

Research tip

Find out more about Acorns hospices. Go to www.acorns.org.uk

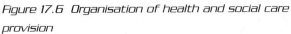

Private and informal

Private provision is paid for directly by the patient at the time. Many older people pay fees to live in a residential care home or to have help at home. Care is also often provided informally, i.e. family members or friends will help with shopping or jobs around the home.

Social services

Social services are services provided by the government at a local level. Health is administered nationally, but social services are administered by your local authority. The Children Act 2004 requires all local authorities to create new accountabilities for children's services. In some areas, social services are now organised under the directorate of Adults and Communities and the directorate of Children, Young People and Families.

Social care services care for vulnerable groups such as children, those families finding it difficult to cope, people with disabilities or mental health problems, or people who have housing or financial problems. They also offer care to some older people.

Many councils work together to run social care services. Often social care services are run jointly with health services, especially when providing services for older people, or those with mental or physical disabilities.

Research tip

Find out what is available in your local area by checking out the local council website link from www.direct.gov.uk

The Commission for Social Care Inspection inspects and regulates all social care providers in England. The Commission also publishes reports on the performance of local councils in delivering social care. The commission's website allows the public to search the directory of care homes and other services in England; and obtain free copies of inspection reports about each care home or service. They also offer advice on choosing a good care home or care service.

Research tip

Check out some care homes in your area by going to the CSCI website www.csci.org.uk

National Health Service (NHS)

The National Health Service is responsible for all health services in England and Wales. Strategic Health Authorities (SHAs) manage the NHS locally and are a key link between the Department of Health and the NHS.

Strategic health authorities (SHAs)

The whole of England is split into 10 strategic health authorities (SHAs). There were originally 28 strategic health authorities (SHAs) but in 2006 this was reduced to 10. Fewer SHAs mean they have stronger commissioning functions, leading to better services for patients and better value for money for taxpayers. One of the functions of SHAs is to commission places for nursing from local universities. The SHA tells the nursing departments how many nurses they need, and the university then offers that number of places.

SHAs develop plans for improving health services in their local area and make sure their local NHS organisations perform well. Within each SHA, the NHS is split into various types of trusts that take responsibility for running the different NHS services in the local area. SHAs are also responsible for making sure national priorities are integrated into local health service plans so, for example, national programmes for improving cancer services are linked to local provision.

There are several different types of trust, as outlined below.

Acute trusts

Acute trusts make sure that hospitals provide high-quality healthcare, and spend their money efficiently. Acute trusts decide how each hospital will develop and improve services. These acute trusts employ nurses, doctors, pharmacists, midwives and health visitors, physiotherapists, radiographers, podiatrists, speech and language therapists, counsellors, occupational therapists and psychologists. They also employ non-medical staff such as receptionists, porters, cleaners, specialists in information technology, managers, engineers, caterers and domestic and security staff.

Increasingly some acute trusts are becoming regional specialist centres. Local hospitals are losing specialist facilities which then go to the regional centre. Regional centres are often linked to universities and become training centres for the nurses and doctors of the future.

Foundation trusts

NHS Foundation Trusts ('foundation hospitals') are a new type of NHS Trust in England. They have power to make decisions on strategy and finance and are more responsive to local needs. Foundation trusts are run by local managers, staff and representatives of the public. They offer services according to the needs of the area, so if there is a high incidence of kidney problems in an area for example, they may develop a specialist renal unit. NHS Foundation Trusts represent a profound change in way in which hospital services are managed. Previously they were managed centrally; now they are being managed locally.

Ambulance trusts

Ambulance trusts provide emergency care such as rapid response teams. In some areas they also provide some transport for patients to get to hospital.

Care trusts

Care trusts work in both health and social care. They carry out a range of services, including social care, mental health services or primary care services. Care trusts are set up when the NHS and local authorities agree to work together, usually where it is felt that a closer relationship between health and social care is needed or would benefit local care services.

Mental health trusts

Mental health trusts provide care for people with mental health problems. They offer counselling in the community and community psychiatric nursing as well as more acute care.

Primary care trusts

Primary care trusts provide the first care. This care may be provided by the the local doctor (GP) or the NHS dentist. Primary care trusts also provide NHS walk-in centres and NHS Direct telephone help. The government puts most of the money for health care into primary care trusts so that local services provide care to meet local needs.

Special health authorities

These include the National Blood Authority, which serves the whole of the country.

Secondary health care

Secondary health care relates to the second type of health care you may receive after you have seen your GP or optician or dentist. It includes hospital and day centre care.

Booked admissions will give patients a choice of appointments and admission dates, speeding up the service for patients. Some hospitals have had to be reorganised to enhance the range of secondary services available locally. Accident and emergency facilities are now centralised at major hospitals where full teams provide a service 24 hours a day. There has been an increase in day surgery and reduced hospital stays for many operations. Some treatments such as minor surgery and diagnostic procedures are now offered at treatment centres.

Some health care is now delivered for the NHS by the private sector. Private hospitals are paid by the NHS to perform investigations and minor surgery to reduce waiting list times. Support workers have been brought in to help radiographers with screening programmes and the use of support workers is being extended in professions allied to medicine.

Integrated care

Care trusts (see above), which were introduced in 2002, are a combination of current NHS and local authority services. Care trusts provide improved customer-focused services which are responsive to local needs. However, in caring for people with learning disabilities, the medical model of care is not always appropriate.

People with learning disabilities now have Learning Disability Partnership Boards and the Valuing People support team as well as the learning Disability Task Force to represent their views. The National Forum for People with Learning Difficulties can influence what happens locally.

The social model of disability is more appropriate for people with learning disabilities. This client group may be disadvantaged by a medical model of care. The Department of Health suggests that care trusts must use a person-centred approach and involve people with learning disabilities as equal partners in decisions which affect them. Partnership with local authorities, Connexions and the other partnerships formed to deliver LD services locally must be maintained.

Integrated care opportunities arise in planning continuing care, tackling delayed hospital discharges or transfers, and pooling money and other resources. The Health Act 1999 allows and encourages resources and management structures to be integrated.

Children's trusts

The Children Act 2004 emerged from the report *Every Child Matters* which in turn followed the enquiry into the death of Victoria Climbie. Children's Trusts bring together all the professionals involved with children so they can work together for the benefit of children in their care. The aim is to break down professional barriers, reduce duplication and improve the service. The Common Assessment framework is used to share information and plan care together so that schools, social workers, doctors and community nurses are all aware of what is being done to help a child.

Accountability for meeting statutory duties is retained but services may be provided differently. Listening to the views of children and young people is an important aspect of children's trusts.

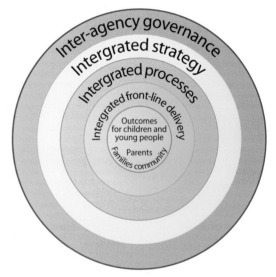

Figure 17.7 Onion Model of children's trusts, commonly referred to as the DFES model.
Source: DFES

SOCIAL CARE SETTINGS AND SERVICES

Since the 1990 NHS and Community Care Act, the role of social workers has changed. Social services departments had originally provided services directly, so there were residential homes and domiciliary carers provided by the state. Since 1990 social workers have had a commissioning role, planning and organising care and then contracting it – mostly from the private sector.

Residential care may be provided by individual care homes run by owner/managers, or the care home might be part of a larger chain of care homes. Domiciliary care, where care is given in the client's own home, is often provided by private care agencies.

Meals on Wheels, offered by the voluntary group WRVS (Women's Royal Voluntary Service), provide a hot or frozen meal delivered to a client's home for a fee. The client must pay for this service. Some local authorities provide this service as Meals Direct but again the client pays for the service.

Home helps are no longer available as a statutory service. Home helps are now part of the private sector of social care. Live-in home helps may charge clients up to £700 per week. They provide social care but do not offer nursing care.

Day care is provided by social services for those people who have been assessed as needing help. Day centres provide a chance to meet other people and take part in different activities. Voluntary organisations often work with social services to provide this care.

Charges are made according to a person's ability to pay and are based on a financial assessment.

Child care may be available from registered childminders, at a playgroup for two hours two or three times a week, or at a nursery. Many private nurseries offer good quality child care provision. Some child care may be offered by local authorities or by Sure Start as statutory provision.

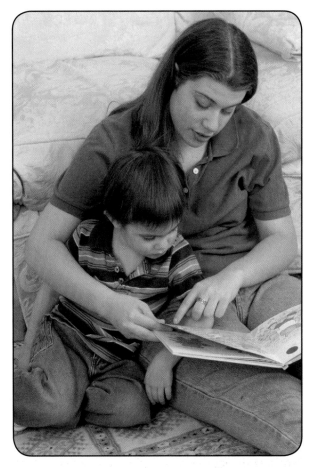

Figure 17.8 Registered childminders provide childcare for many families

Foster care is needed when children cannot be cared for by their own parents. This can be for many different reasons and different types of foster care are offered according to the needs of both the child and their family. There is short-term care from a few days to a few weeks, long-term placements, and also care for disabled children or children with behavioural problems.

There are different types of foster care: emergency care provides a safe place to stay for a short time. Other types include long-term care, short-term care, or short breaks. Sometimes special foster care is arranged when a young person is on remand or for children who need specialist care. Sometimes family members care for a child until the parents can cope.

Research tip

The following link will help you find what sort of child care is available in your area: www.childcarelink.gov.uk/index.asp

ACCESS TO SOCIAL CARE SERVICES

Referral

A person or a child may be referred to social care services by a professional such as a doctor, or in the case of a child, by a teacher. Sometimes a concerned neighbour may make the referral. Occasionally a person self refers. It might be an older person who asks for help, or it may be a child who rings Childline for help.

After referral, the social worker makes an assessment. In the case of a child this may be done in an emergency situation and the child might not have much choice, as the social worker has a duty of care to the child and a legal obligation to provide a safe environment for the child. Older people may have a more equal part to play in the assessment, and more choice in what care to accept.

Barriers to access

Barriers to access may be geographical, for example, one local authority might offer a service which is not available in another area. Individual preference may prevent people getting a service. Many older people do not claim benefits because they feel it is a matter of pride to be independent. Financially a person may be asset-rich and cash-poor, for example, they may live in a large house worth a lot of money but have very little cash to live on. They may not wish to move from a familiar place to a strange home.

There may be social barriers to access as some families support each other and do not like to ask for help. This may throw a heavy burden on relatives. There may be cultural barriers as some older people expect to live with their married sons and do not think to ask for help from social care services. Individuals may also have specific needs, for example, they may not speak English, and may not wish to attend a day centre where they cannot understand others. They may be visually impaired and perhaps there are no facilities to meet their needs.

CHILDREN AND YOUNG PEOPLE

Every Child Matters (2003) was the government response to the death of Victoria Climbié. It focused on the care of children and young people from birth to age 19. The government's aim is for every child to have the support they need to:

- Be healthy

- Stay safe

- Enjoy and achieve

- Make a positive contribution

- Achieve economic well-being.

Joint working between hospitals, schools, police and voluntary groups will ensure sharing of information to protect children and young people from harm. Children and young people should have a voice in what happens to them. Integrated services, children's trusts, consisting of local authorities and partners will work together and involve children when planning. A Children's Commissioner for England was appointed in 2005, to give children and young people a voice.

The Children's Fund identifies children and young people at risk of social exclusion, and makes sure they receive the support they need.

A Common Assessment Framework (CAF) provides a national, common process for early assessment to identify all the child's individual, family and community needs, which can be built up over time and shared between practitioners. A common process reduces duplication and streamlines assessment.

Extended schooling is a way of delivering the outcomes for *Every Child Matters* and aims to improve attendance and achievement. An extended school works with local providers, agencies (and other schools) to provide a core of integrated services:

- wraparound childcare all year round (in primary schools)

- parenting and family support

- activities including study support, sport and music clubs

- easy referral to specialist services such as health and social care

- community use of facilities, including adult and family learning and ICT.

England, Wales, Northern Ireland and Scotland vary in provision of care.

EVIDENCE ACTIVITY

P2

P2 Describe the overall structure of social care service provision in home country.

You are the public relations officer for a local council and need to describe the overall structure of social care provision in your own country to introduce an item for the council newsletter. You may use labelled diagrams to help you explain the overall structure.

17.3 Understand roles and responsibilities in the social care sector

OVERARCHING ORGANISATIONS

Roles and responsibilities

The Department of Health has overall responsibility for health and social care. In England, social care services are provided largely by local councils. Social care services also tackle social exclusion nationally and locally. Both social services and the NHS are being modernised in an effort to raise standards of care, improve the experiences of service users and reduce duplication.

Social care organisations are shown in the diagram below:

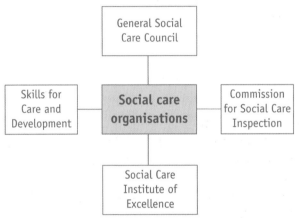

Figure 17.9 Social care organisations

General Social Care Council/Care Council for Wales/Northern Ireland Social Care Council

> **Think** Did you know that: The Department of Health is the General Social Care Council's sponsoring Government department? Care Council for Wales (CCW) is the General Social Care Council's equivalent body in Wales? Northern Ireland Social Care Council (NISCC) is the General Social Care Council's equivalent body in Northern Ireland? Scottish Social Services Council (SSSC) is the General Social Care Council's equivalent body in Scotland?

The General Social Care Council (GSCC) regulates and maintains standards for the social care workforce. The GSCC was established in 2001 as part of the Care Standards Act 2000. The three main functions of the GSCC are to:

- establish codes of practice for social care workers and employers

- set up a register of social care workers in England

- regulate social work education and training.

All qualified social workers must register with the GSCC. Other workers will register later.

There are two codes of practice:

- The Code of Practice for Social Care Workers sets out the standards of professional conduct and practice required of social care workers.

- The Code of Practice for Employers of Social Care Workers sets out the responsibilities of employers in regulating social care workers.

The codes of practice provide a guide for those who work in social care, setting out the standards of conduct that workers and their employers should meet. Service users, carers and the wider public know what standard of conduct and practice to expect from these codes.

'Regulation' means that the GSCC can decide who is allowed to work in social care. The conduct process allows the GSCC to take action and investigate complaints against social workers. Social workers who breach the Code of Practice for Social Care Workers could be removed from the register through this process. An interim suspension order suspends the social worker from the Social Care Register temporarily until the complaint is investigated. The individual will not be able to work as a social worker until a full conduct hearing has been held and they have been cleared.

> **Think** Why do we need a common code of conduct for all social care workers?

Research tip

Find out more about the General Social Care Council from their website: www.gscc.org.uk

Skills for Care and Development

Skills for Care and Development is the Sector Skills Council for social care, children and young people's workforces in the UK. It is made up of five organisations: Care Council for Wales, Children's Workforce Development Council, Northern Ireland Social Care Council, Scottish Social Services Council, and Skills for Care.

Skills for Care and Development (SfC&D) is licensed by the government to represent the interests of social care employers and workers across the UK. A range of both public authorities and independent organisations is commissioned by the public sector to deliver social care services but sometimes they act directly for people who receive the services.

Employers want appropriately skilled and qualified workers. The Sector Skills Council has worked with service users and carers, education and training providers, national stakeholders and the health sector to achieve this. The Sector Skills Council also worked with awarding bodies to produce the new Specialist Diploma so that the qualification meets the needs of employers.

Research tip

You can find out more about the work of the Sector Skills Council on www.skillsforcareanddevelopment.org.uk

The Commission for Social Care Inspection (CSCI)

The CSCI registers, inspects and reports on adult social care services in England in order to improve social care and get rid of bad practice.

Research tip

Look at the website for the CSCI www.csci.org.uk/. You can read an inspection report for your local care home or make a complaint about poor quality care.

Children's services are inspected by Ofsted.

CSCI inspect local councils too. The type and frequency of inspection varies. There are three types of inspection:

- Key inspections look at how well a service is doing, taking into account information provided by the owner or manager and taking into account any complaints. Service users and their relatives may be asked their views too. Inspectors see if the care given meets the standards set by the government. Key inspections are unannounced, which means they do not tell the care provider they are coming to inspect.

- Random inspections are short, targeted inspections that focus on specific issues or check that recommendations have been carried out. Random inspections are also used to investigate complaints. They are unannounced and can take place at any time of day or night.

- Thematic inspections look at specific issues, such as medication or infection control, and may look at trends in certain areas. CSCI produce reports based on these findings.

Social Care Institute of Excellence (SCIE)

The SCIE develops and promotes knowledge about good practice in the sector. SCIE shares resources to help social care workers and service users.

Research tip

You can find reports, knowledge reviews and position papers on a variety of topics relating to social care on the website: www.scie.org.uk

Social care online is a website set up by SCIE to provide easy-to-find information on topics such as benefits, pensions, housing and social policy.

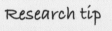

Research tip

You may find this website useful when you need to research a topic for an assignment. Go to: www.scie-socialcareonline.org.uk

REGULATION

As explained above, the General Social Care Council/Care Council for Wales/Northern Ireland regulates the workforce, providing Social Care Council codes of practice for workers and for employers.

> ***Think*** What is different and what is the same when you compare the employer's code of conduct and the social care worker's code of conduct? How does each code improve social care service provision?

Role of Sector Skills Councils

There are 25 Sector Skills Councils (SSCs). Each SSC covers a specific sector of employment in the UK and is led by employers. They are licensed by the government but are independent so they do not have to do what the government wants. This is the way employers can influence government policy and education services so that the skills they need in their workers are taught. SSCs aim to reduce skills shortages, improve the productivity of the workforce and increase the amount of training workers receive.

The Sector Skills Council for Care and Development covers social care, children and young people.

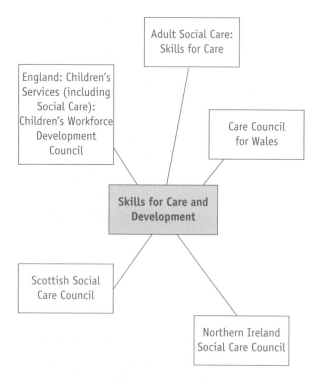

Figure 17.10 The Sector Skills Council for Care and Development is an umbrella organisation

EVIDENCE ACTIVITY

P3, M2

P3 Describe the roles and responsibilities of three overarching organisations in social care.

M2 Explain the roles of the three organisations in improving social care provision.

As press officer for the council you time the newsletter to be distributed a week before the next local elections. You wish to inform readers about three overarching organisations in the social care sector but you have to assume your audience knows little about the organisations, their roles or responsibilities.

Your article needs to describe the roles and responsibilities of three overarching organisations in the social care sector. Again your audience will appreciate diagrams or pictures to support your description. 'Overarching' means 'being part of the big picture' so you will need three large providers. 'Roles' are what the organisations do. Responsibilities include who they are responsible to. You may like to use a table to help your audience understand each section:

	Roles	Responsible to
Organisation 1		
Organisation 2		
Organisation 3		

You anticipate some opposition at the election and want to show the public how these organisations have improved social care provision, so you draft a leaflet to be handed to each person as they arrive. The leaflet will need an eye-catching title and should explain the roles of the three organisations in improving social care service provision (M2).

LEGISLATION, STANDARDS AND CODES OF PRACTICE

Care Standards Act 2000

The Care Standards Act 2000 is a major piece of legislation. Some of the key points of this act were to:

- establish a National Care Standards Commission

- register and regulate children's homes, independent hospitals and clinics, care homes, residential family centres, independent medical agencies, domiciliary care agencies, fostering agencies, nurses agencies and voluntary adoption agencies

- ensure that local authority fostering and adoption services are regulated and inspected

- establish a General Social Care Council and a Care Council for Wales

- make provision for the registration, regulation and training of social care workers

- establish a Children's Commissioner for Wales

- ensure that childminders and providers of day care are registered, regulated and trained

- provide for the protection of children and vulnerable adults

- amend the law about children looked after in schools and colleges

- repeal the Nurses Agencies Act 1957

- amend Schedule 1 to the Local Authority Social Services Act 1970.

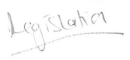

Research tip

You can read more about the Care Standards Act on the government website www.opsi.gov.uk

Children Act 2004

The Children Act 2004 came about after the government published a green paper, *Every Child Matters*, for consultation in 2003. This was in itself a response to a formal inquiry after the failure of social and health services led to the horrific death of Victoria Climbie at the hands of her aunt. Legislation for supporting services to children and young people was then revised and brought together under the Children Act 2004.

Part 1 of the Act provides for the establishment of a Children's Commissioner to make sure that children and young people have a means of being heard in England, Northern Ireland, Wales and Scotland. Part 2 of the Act supports integrated planning, commissioning, and delivery of children's services and provides for clear accountability.

The Act requires local authorities to make arrangements for key agencies to co-operate to improve the well-being of children and young people and widen pool budgets in support of this. It establishes statutory Local Safeguarding Children Boards to replace the existing non-statutory Area Child Protection Committees. Children's services authorities must publish a Children and Young People's Plan (CYPP) which will set out their strategy for services for children and relevant young people. The Act allows the creation of databases holding information on all children and young people in order to facilitate joint working.

Part 2 ensures clear accountability for children's services. Local authorities in England must appoint a director of children's services to be accountable for the local authority's education and social services functions in so far as they relate to children. There must be an integrated inspection framework for joint reviews of all children's services provided in an area. There is a new duty for local authorities to promote the educational achievement of looked after children.

Part 1 of the Act, which establishes the Commissioner, covers the United Kingdom. Part 2 is concerned only with England and Part 3 only with Wales.

National minimum standards

National minimum standards say what a minimum level of service is. They are guidelines for good practice to help inspectors judge the standard of service across care. There are National Minimum Standards for Care homes for older people, for care homes with adult placements, for care homes for adults aged 18-25, for nurses agencies, domiciliary care and for adult placement schemes. Children's services are inspected by Ofsted.

National occupational standards

Occupational standards describe the skills, knowledge and understanding needed to undertake a particular task or job to a nationally recognised level of competence. Some of the competences for social work include:

- prepare for social work contact and involvement

- work with individuals, families, carers, groups and communities to help them make informed decisions

- interact with individuals, families, carers, groups and communities to achieve change and development and to improve life opportunities.

Research tip

You can see the occupational standards for a chosen job on www.ukstandards.org

Organisational policies and procedures

Organisational policies and procedures are drawn from key legislation, charters and codes of practice. As well as covering legal requirements for anti-discriminatory practice and health and safety, policies will govern joint working arrangements in the changing world of health care.

ACCOUNTABILITIES

Accountabilities to professional bodies have already been mentioned but there is also accountability to the line manager when employed. At times there may be conflict; for example, if a manager asks a social worker to work when staffing levels are inadequate. The first duty of care is to the client and the professional must always remember that they alone are accountable for their work. A disciplinary hearing will not accept the plea that 'a manager told me to do it'. Professionals are accountable for their own practice.

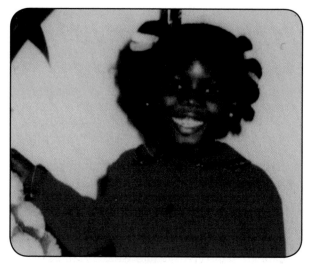

Figure 17.11 Victoria Climbie

In the Victoria Climbie case, the social worker and her manager were both dismissed for gross misconduct. The General Social Care council would now hold a disciplinary hearing for any complaints made against social workers.

REDRESS

There are procedures for complaints both internally and externally. Trade unions usually have local representatives who will accompany members to hearings. In some cases professional associations are the regulatory bodies and may conduct their own hearings in a case of alleged misconduct. 'Whistle blowing', or reporting of bad practice, is a last resort to be used if all else fails. It must be done sensitively to protect patients.

LEADERSHIP AND MANAGEMENT

The General Social Care Council regulates and supports social work education and training. They accredit the universities that offer undergraduate and post-qualifying social work qualifications and quality-approve social work courses. Once qualified, a social worker has to keep up to date, completing 90 hours of continuing professional development over three years in order to maintain registration.

The Code of Practice for Employers of Social Care Workers states that employers must support registered workers to meet continuing professional development requirements that are consistent with their work and the aims of the employer. Supervision sessions with employers should identify areas for personal development, identify training and learning needs, develop and monitor the training and learning plan and make changes where necessary. This is often part of the appraisal process.

Self-employed social workers must also meet the requirements for post-registration training in order to renew their registration.

Employers must offer induction and monitor the performance of individuals. Social care workers who are not qualified social workers will be expected to work towards National Vocational Qualifications. Employers are expected to provide leadership, build effective teams and allocate tasks appropriately. Different social work environments will interpret this differently, so in a local authority, leadership and guidance will come from the senior management. In a care home, leadership and management may come from the manager. In both cases, care workers must be trained and have clearly defined responsibilities.

ROLE OF WORKFORCE DEVELOPMENT

The Children's Workforce Development Council (CWDC) covers:

- nursery workers
- daycare workers
- childminders
- nannies
- education welfare
- learning mentors
- Connexions advisors
- foster care
- children and family social workers
- children's home staff
- CAFCASS (Children and Family Court Advisory and Support Service).

CWDC is led by employers to make sure that anyone who works with children has the right training so they can work together for the best interests of the children. CWDC is a member of the UK Skills for Care and Development, which is part of the sector skills council.

Skills for Care ensure that qualifications and standards meet the needs of people who use care services. They develop national standards and a qualification framework for the sector, collect data and research issues affecting carers and people who use care services, create a national plan for workforce development, and enable employers to work jointly with health, local government and education at local, regional and national level.

Skills for Care regional committees work in their own region of the country. Most members are from employers in the independent and statutory sectors. Other members are service users and carers, staff groups and training interests.

Funding

There are many sources of funding and one of the most difficult tasks is making sure all funding for training is used.

Research tip

Find out more about funding –
www.topssengland.net

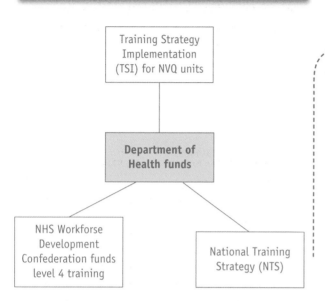

Figure 17.12 *Sources of funding for training*

Training strategy implementation (TSI) funding pays for staff training for employers. There is a limit to the amount of funding. The National Training Strategy (NTS) gives money to local authorities to pay for staff training in private, voluntary and statutory sectors. The NHS Workforce Development Confederation pays for staff to undertake a level 4 qualification linked to their job role if they do not already have this.

Money comes from the European Social Fund and from the government to the Learning and Skills Council to pay for NVQs and apprenticeships and to support employers through Business Link.

There are also government schemes for individuals. Apprenticeships are funded through the Learning and Skills Council: there are Young Apprenticeships (14-16 year olds) and Apprenticeships (16-24 year olds), as well as Adult Apprenticeships for learners over the age of 25. Entry to Employment is an entry to Level 1 programmes for those young people not yet ready for an apprenticeship. New Deal provides return to work programmes.

WORKING IN TEAMS

Working in teams, particularly in joint teams where people come from different professional backgrounds, can place many demands on workers. Individuals may have so many differing needs and requirements to be met.

Example

Dave uses heroin and, when he needs a fix, he robs older ladies of their handbags to get the money to feed his drug habit. At a joint meeting, a social worker may be concerned with Dave's social needs, such as the fact that he lives in a squat. A nurse may be concerned with his health needs, and the risk of him getting HIV from sharing used needles. A youth and community justice representative may be concerned with the effect he has on those he steals from.

The needs of individuals within a multi-disciplinary team come together in a holistic approach, where the client is the focus of care, rather than the service. Methods of working are changing to include other professionals, partly as a result of legislation such as the Children Act 2004, and the Care Standards Act 2000. Training of social care workers now includes joint working and sharing good practice across sectors.

EVIDENCE ACTIVITY

P4, M3

P4 Describe three examples of legislation, policies, standards or codes of practice that influence social care service provision.

M3 Explain the role of legislation, policies, standards or codes of practice in improving social care service provision.

You are to prepare an induction pack for new staff to show three examples of how legislation, policies, standards or codes of practice influence provision of social care services. You will need to explain in the pack how each example has improved the provision of these services. New staff may be from any job role in social services so the pack must be easily understood by all.

EVIDENCE ACTIVITY

P5, D1

Part of your role involves working in the human resources department. Your boss asks you to prepare a presentation to (1) explain the role of workforce development in the social care sector (P5) and (2) evaluate the requirements of social care workers in terms of providing a competent workforce in social care services (D1).

17.4 *Understand multi-disciplinary working in the social care sector*

Every Child Matters shows there are three main ways of delivering multi-agency services: a multi-agency panel, a multi-agency team and an integrated service.

EXAMPLES OF WORKING IN PARTNERSHIP

Examples of partnership working may be seen in Children's Trusts where multi-agency working puts the service users at the heart of planning and decision making.

In the health service, a psychiatric unit for adolescents may have a team of doctors, nurses, psychologists, occupational therapists, a family therapist, an art therapist, teachers and social workers. The social worker may not work with all the young people admitted but may work with those with accommodation needs, or social needs, and those with child protection issues, helping them to get ready for the time when they will no longer be in-patients. The social worker may advise others in the team on child protection issues, and referrals to social services, and may contribute directly to the care of young people by organising carers' meetings or user-involvement groups.

Links with the NHS may be forged through joint working in the community. An example from practice of joint working is a Community Mental Health Team for older adults and those with dementia. Community mental health nurses, occupational therapists and social workers make up the team.

Higher Education Institutions (HEIs) are required by government to involve service users and carers in the design and delivery of social work training. An example from practice shows how this can happen: the University of East Anglia developed a placement assessment form, a monitoring form, and a student and service user feedback form tools to monitor practice learning.

Research tip

Find out more by going to
www.scie.org.uk

The case study adapted from the Every Child Matters website below, shows multi-agency working between the probation service, youth offending team, education service and the health and social care teams.

CASE STUDY: CONNEXIONS REFERRAL TO MIDWIFERY

Martha was 15 and pregnant. She met the Specialist Connexions PA at a sexual health drop-in. The PA provided support, including telling her family and seeing her GP. Martha chose to continue with the pregnancy and met the Teenage Pregnancy Midwife who provided antenatal care. Martha had stopped attending school some time before and she was on probation. The multi-agency team worked closely with Martha and Social Care to ensure she was assessed on her own merit. At first, Social Care had planned to take Martha's baby into care at birth. The Teenage Pregnancy team acted as advocate and it was agreed that Social Care would provide a joint foster placement for mum and baby. Multi-agency meetings were also arranged for Martha with the Education and the Youth Offending Service. The TP team helped Martha become proactive in planning her and her baby's future. The Specialist Connexions PA liaised with the school to ensure Martha received some education during the pregnancy.

Outcome: Martha and her baby remain together in foster care. All professionals involved comment on what a good mother Martha is. Martha is also attending college and her baby receives childcare in the college, which is paid for with Care to Learn support for childcare costs.

Extended schooling

Extended schooling should be available to all children by 2010. This includes study support activities such as homework, sports and music clubs, with childcare available from 8am to 6pm all year round, and parenting programmes and family learning sessions to allow children to learn with their parents. Children with particular needs will be referred quickly to specialist support services such as speech therapy, child and adolescent mental health services, family support services, intensive behaviour support and sexual health services. There will be ICT, sports and arts facilities, and adult learning for the wider community. One in five schools already provides extended services in partnership with voluntary, private and independent providers.

Extended services benefit schools by improving pupil attainment, reducing exclusion rates and building self-confidence, which in turn improves relationships and produces better attitudes to learning. Parents benefit as extended childcare allows flexible working. Extended services reduce barriers to learning.

Schools work in partnership with local private and voluntary sector providers, or work with other schools to offer the services. Local authorities are key partners in developing extended schools. There is close local cooperation between partners working in education, childcare, children's centres, health and other children's services.

ContinYou and 4Children - both charitable organisations - support the extended schools agenda. ContinYou provides technical support through the Extended Schools Support Service, including advice on health improvement, community regeneration and study support. 4Children provides advice on childcare linked to extended schools, including delivery models and quality assurance programmes.

Over 800 children aged up to 13 years old use the childcare provision offered by Franche First Primary School, Kidderminister, Worcestershire. There are holiday and term-time play schemes, play activities, out-of-school clubs and activities to involve parents in their children's education and lifelong learning opportunities.

THE PURPOSE OF WORKING IN PARTNERSHIP

A holistic approach benefits all. Partners identify common aims and objectives with the child or client. This approach promotes integration, reduces duplication, maximises resources and ensures a consistent approach which is especially important where people are vulnerable. Working in partnership benefits everyone as a more efficient skill mix of staff may be allocated to provide the best possible care at the least cost to the tax payer.

Figure 17.13 SureStart is an example of joint working

EVIDENCE ACTIVITY

P6, M4, D2

P6 Describe two examples of multi-disciplinary working in social care.

M4 Explain how multi-disciplinary working can improve social care provision.

D2 Use examples to evaluate the effectiveness of multi-disciplinary working for service users.

You are hoping for an early night but a colleague goes off sick and you are asked to step in to explain multi-disciplinary working in the social care sector to the local council tomorrow. You need to prepare a talk which lasts for about five minutes and you will need to provide notes so your colleague knows what you said in their absence.

The talk must: describe two examples of multi-disciplinary working in social care; explain how multi-disciplinary working can improve social care provision and use examples to evaluate the effectiveness of multi-disciplinary working for service users.

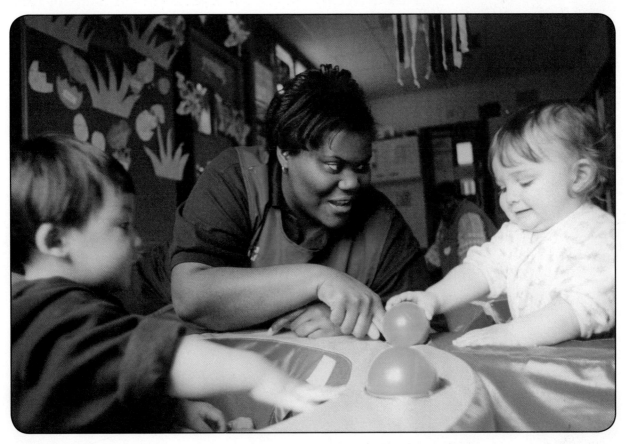

in the Health Sector

Unit 18

This unit helps you to find out about working in the health sector and the current organisation and administration of health care. It provides preparation for a career in health care by explaining the personal qualities as well as the training and qualifications needed to work in this sector.

This unit is particularly useful if combined with a health care placement for Unit 6 and Units 44 or 45.

This unit may not be combined in a programme with Unit 18: Working in the Social Care Sector.

Learning outcomes

On completion of this unit you will be able to:

So, you want to be a...

Physiotherapist

My name Angela Meiklem
Age 25
Income £22,000

If you are looking for a hands on role with a lot of variety and great career prospects, read on, this could be the job for you.

What do you do?

I assess and treat people using movement and exercise, manipulation, massage and hydrotherapy. I treat a variety of people such as post operative patients, people with respiratory problems and orthopaedic patients. I advise patients and carers on how to prevent and manage health problems.

I sometimes attend case conferences, and help to manage the caseload as well as maintaining records. I work within the NHS which makes for a busy environment with plenty of variety. I find working as part of a multidisciplinary team very satisfying.

How did you become a Physiotherapist?

I have a B.Sc. (Hons) degree in Physiotherapy; this is the most common route into the profession. I gained some experience working as a physiotherapy assistant which was a great advantage when it came to interviews. Physiotherapy is a competitive area, so it helps to have something extra to show your commitment.

Once you have qualified you need to register with the Health Professions Council in order to work as a physiotherapist and membership of the Chartered Society of Physiotherapists is also recommended.

> **I work within the NHS which makes for a busy environment with plenty of variety**

What skills does a physiotherapist need?

Good communication skills are essential in this job, you must be able to work well with other professionals and be able to build rapport with patients. You will be working very closely with patients so you need to be able to get along with a lot of different types of people. Strong organisational abilities and good time management are also needed.

What's the pay like?

I started on around £19,000 and this will rise to about £24,000 as I gain more experience. Team leaders can earn up to £36,000 and Consultants up to £88,000.

What are the hours like?

Usually it is the standard 9 to 5 but there may be some occasional weekend or evening work.

What are your plans for the future?

I would like to set up my own private practice and become self employed.

Grading criteria

The table shows what you need to do to gain a pass, merit or distinction in this part of the qualification. Make sure you refer back to it when you are completing work so you can judge whether you are meeting the criteria and what you need to do to fill in gaps in your knowledge or experience.

In this unit there are five evidence activities that give you an opportunity to demonstrate your achievement of the grading criteria.

page 143	P1, M1		page 154	P4, P5, M3, D1
page 151	P2		page 155	P6, M4, D2
page 153	P3, M2			

To achieve a pass grade the evidence must show that the learner is able to...	To achieve a merit grade the evidence must show that, in addition to the pass criteria, the learner is able to...	To achieve a distinction grade the evidence must show that, in addition to the pass and merit criteria, the learner is able to...
P1 Describe the requirements for two careers in the health sector	**M1** Explain how the requirements of health care workers can contribute to providing a positive experience for patients	**D1** Evaluate the requirements of health care workers in terms of providing a competent workforce for the health sector
P2 Describe the overall structure of health services provision in home country		
P3 Describe the roles and responsibilities of three overarching organisations in the health sector	**M2** Explain the roles of the three organisations in improving health services provision	
P4 Describe three examples of legislation, policies, standards or codes of practice that influence provision of health services	**M3** Explain the role of legislation, policies, standards or codes of practice in improving provision of health services	
P5 Explain the role of workforce development in the health sector		
P6 Describe two examples of multi-disciplinary working in the health sector.	**M4** Explain how multi-disciplinary working can improve the provision of health services.	**D2** Use examples to evaluate the effectiveness of multi-disciplinary working for patients.

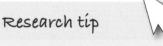

18.1 Understand potential careers in the health sector

There are many different careers in the health sector. Not everyone wants to be a nurse or a doctor. We also need physiotherapists, radiographers and laboratory technicians.

CAREER FRAMEWORK FOR HEALTH

Health workers have many valuable skills, such as being able to work with others, and communicating effectively with different people. In the past, health workers who wanted to develop their careers moved on from the health service into other jobs, such as teaching or management, and their skills were lost to the health care workforce. Government policy now aims to keep such people in the health workforce by offering career development. According to the Career Framework for Health, shown below, someone could start at the bottom, on level 1, with few skills and work up to level 9, a senior position, by increasing their skills and knowledge through learning and development. This is called skills escalation, or skills improvement. It will meet workforce needs in the NHS and help people to develop their careers without leaving the health service. Non-clinical and managerial roles do not as yet fit into the framework.

Table 18.1 Career framework for health

Level	Job
9	More senior staff
8	Consultant practitioners
7	Advanced practitioners
6	Senior practitioners/specialist practitioners
5	Practitioners
4	Assistant practitioners/associate practitioners
3	Senior healthcare assistants/ technicians
2	Support workers
1	Initial entry jobs

Research tip

Read more about skills escalation on www.skillsforhealth.org.uk

POTENTIAL CAREERS

There are many potential careers in the health sector. Some involve professional training full time at university. Others involve part-time study or on-the-job training. The NHS Careers website lists many different health careers.

Research tip

This website will help you to find out more about different careers in the health service: www.nhscareers.nhs.uk/

Medicine and dentistry are both health careers. Professions allied to medicine include dieticians, occupational therapists, radiographers and many more.

Dentistry

Dentists care for the teeth and gums. They work in hospital or community settings. Dentists are regulated by the General Dental Council which protects patients and regulates the dental team.

Dental nurses work with and support the dentist. They get instruments ready, mix materials and make patients comfortable.

Dental hygienists carry out scaling and polishing of teeth. They apply topical fluoride and fissure sealants to teeth.

All dental technicians, nurses and dental hygienists must also register as Dental Care Professionals with the General Dental Council by 31 July 2008.

Research tip

Follow this link www.gdc-uk.org to find out more about the General Dental Council.

Medicine

You need good A-level results, usually in sciences, in order to train as a doctor at a medical school attached to a university. It is hard to become a medical student as many more people apply than there are places available. The course lasts for five years, during which time students have increasing contact with patients in a variety of settings. Medical students are attached to GP surgeries and work in community health in areas such as psychiatry and sexual health. They also have placements in hospitals on medical and surgical wards. Once a doctor is qualified they work as a house officer, usually on a rotational job, for a further two years. They then specialise in one area of medicine and have to study for a specialist qualification as a surgeon, physician, psychiatrist or general practitioner.

Doctors must register with the General Medical Council (GMC) to practise medicine in the UK. The GMC regulates doctors which mean they investigate any complaints against a doctor, and issue guidelines for practice.

NURSING AND MIDWIFERY

Nursing and midwifery are regulated by the Nursing and Midwifery Council (NMC). All nurses and midwives must register with the NMC in order to practise and any complaints against nurses or midwives are investigated by the NMC. The NMC issues guidelines for practice and a code of practice which all registered nurses and midwives must follow.

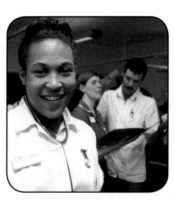

Figure 18.1 A nurse

Research tip

Find out more about the NMC by going to www.nmc-uk.org/

A career in nursing starts with a three-year training at university to study either a diploma or a degree. Both take the same length of time and enable the successful student to register as a nurse, but the funding is different. Currently, those applying to study the diploma at university apply through the Nursing and Midwifery Admissions Service NMAS. Successful applicants are awarded a bursary which they do not have to pay back. Those applying for a nursing degree must apply through UCAS, the Universities and Colleges Admissions Service. Successful applicants for the nursing degree receive a student loan which they must pay back when they graduate. It is currently possible to study for a diploma in nursing and qualify as a nurse, then 'top up' to a degree by taking extra modules after qualifying.

Research tip

Find out more about NMAS. Go to www.nmas.ac.uk

Nursing has four branches – as shown in the diagram below.

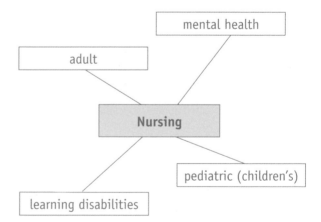

Figure 18.2 There are four areas or branches of nursing

The adult nursing branch equips nurses to work within both hospital and community settings involving preventative, curative and palliative nursing interventions.

Key words

palliative – a drug or medical treatment that reduces pain without curing the cause of the pain

Children's nursing provides the foundation skills needed to nurse children and their families, progressing to subjects such as caring for children and adolescents in hospital, and children with complex and specialised care needs.

Learning disability nursing involves helping individuals to have the same rights, choices, opportunities and life chances that are available to non-disabled individuals in society. This involves assisting individuals with a learning disability to have the opportunity to meet their social, physical, intellectual, cultural, emotional and spiritual needs.

The mental health nursing branch concentrates on caring for people with mental health problems, from caring for adults in crisis to supporting recovery and rehabilitation.

Specialist community public health nurses are also regulated by the NMC. They are qualified nurses who have taken further qualifications in order to work in the community.

Midwives

Midwives are not nurses but are specialists in the care of women and their families and give support, care and advice during pregnancy, labour and the postnatal period. Midwives hand over care to a specialist public health nurse ten days after delivery of the baby.

In the UK, midwives may work alone as independent professionals in the community and in stand-alone birth centres. Fewer midwives now work as independent professionals because the cost of their professional insurance has risen enormously. Midwives are also employed within the NHS, or within private health care.

In the UK midwifery training programmes are offered at universities. The course lasts for three years, but nurses who are already qualified in the adult branch of nursing may fast track on an 18-month programme. At least half the training takes place in clinical practice which may be in hospitals, midwife-led units, birth centres, health centres or the patient's own home.

Midwives care for women with normal uncomplicated pregnancies. Pregnant women with any complications are referred to a gynaecologist. Midwives promote and facilitate normal childbirth and teach health education. Midwives are taught when to call for help and how to recognise emergency situations, respond appropriately and work as part of a team.

Professions allied to medicine

The Health Professions Council registers 13 different health professions allied to medicine:

- art therapists
- biomedical scientists
- chiropodists/podiatrists
- clinical scientists
- occupational therapists
- dieticians
- operating department practitioners
- paramedics
- orthoptists
- physiotherapists
- prosthetists and orthotists
- radiographers
- speech and language therapists.

Dietetics

Dieticians work with people to promote nutritional wellbeing, prevent food-related problems and treat disease. They help patients plan a healthy diet, and work with patients who may have problems such as diabetes or renal failure to plan a diet to help manage their illness. The British Dietetic Association (BDA) is the professional association for dieticians and aims to promote training and education in dietetics. Dieticians also register with the Health Professions Council.

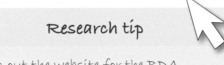

Research tip

Check out the website for the BDA
www.bda.uk.com

Occupational therapy

Occupational therapists (OTs) design programmes of treatment for people who need help to live independently. For example, OTs may organise a ramp for an individual to get in and out of their home, or they may work with someone who has had a brain injury and needs to learn to dress themselves.

OTs work in a variety of settings, including NHS and private hospitals, a person's own home, GP practices, social services departments, charities and voluntary agencies and also housing departments. They specialise in helping people with stress and anxiety, mental health issues, such as eating disorders, rehabilitation following strokes, cardiac problems and accidents. They help people with assistive technology such as mobility aids. They work with community teams and community mental health teams.

The British Association of Occupational Therapists (BAOT) is the professional body and trade union for occupational therapy staff in the UK. The College of Occupational Therapists is part of BAOT and sets professional and educational standards for occupational therapy. It also provides guidance to members but does not regulate their conduct.

Pharmacy

The pharmacist is an expert in medicines. A pharmacist can be involved in any aspect of the preparation and use of medicines, from the discovery of their active ingredients to their use by patients. Pharmacists also monitor the effects of medicines, both for patient care and for research purposes.

To become a pharmacist students study for a four-year masters degree in pharmacy from a school of pharmacy at university, then have one year's practical training in a community or hospital pharmacy and have to pass a registration exam.

The Royal Pharmaceutical Society of Great Britain (RPSGB) is the professional and regulatory body for pharmacists in England, Scotland and Wales. It also regulates pharmacy technicians. The Society regulates and represents the profession of pharmacy.

Research tip

You can find out more on www.pharmacycareers.org.uk/ and about the profession generally on www.rpsgb.org/.

Physiotherapy

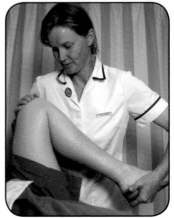

Physiotherapists help and treat people of all ages with physical problems caused by illness, accident or ageing. They see human movement as central to the health and well-being of individuals. Physiotherapists maximise movement

Figure 18.3 A physiotherapist

potential through health promotion, preventive healthcare, treatment and rehabilitation. Physiotherapists use manual therapy, therapeutic exercise and other treatments. They also have an understanding of psychological, cultural and social factors which influence people's health.

Physiotherapists work in hospital outpatients, intensive care, orthopaedic departments and on many wards in hospitals. They also work with children. Physiotherapy can be vital for those with cystic fibrosis. Physios also work in the community where they may be employed by primary care trusts. They may work in a patient's home, in nursing homes or day centres, in schools and in health centres.

All physiotherapists working within the NHS are registered with the regulatory body for physiotherapists: the Health Professions Council (or HPC). Some physiotherapists work in private practice. Unless they are chartered or registered they may not be governed by the code of conduct. The Chartered Society of Physiotherapy is the professional body for chartered physiotherapists, physiotherapy students and assistants.

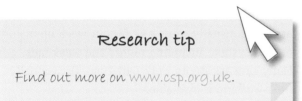

Research tip

Find out more on www.csp.org.uk.

Speech and language therapy

A speech and language therapist (SLT) assesses and treats speech, language and communication problems in people of all ages to enable them to communicate to the best of their ability. A speech and language therapist works directly with clients and their families and works closely with teachers and health professionals, including doctors, nurses and psychologists.

SLTs help children and adults who may have difficulty producing and using speech, difficulty understanding or using language, difficulty with feeding, chewing or swallowing. They work with people who stammer or have voice problems. They also work with people who may have had a stroke, cancer of the mouth and throat, head injury or hearing loss and deafness. They work with people with physical and / or learning disability, dementia and psychiatric disorders. SLTs work in a variety of settings, such as hospitals (both inpatients and outpatients), community

health centres, mainstream and special schools, assessment units and day centres and they also work in clients' homes.

Most speech and language therapy students study a three or four year honours degree at university in the UK. Courses include a balance of theory and practice. There is an accelerated course for those with an appropriate first degree. The Health Professions Council regulates the courses. Students who graduate from these programmes may apply for registration with the Health Professions Council.

Paramedics

Paramedics are often the first healthcare professionals on the scene of any accident or medical emergency. They are usually the senior member of a two-person ambulance crew, with an ambulance technician to help them. Sometimes they work alone, using a motorbike, emergency response car or even a bicycle to reach their patients. With extra training, they can become members of an air ambulance crew.

When paramedics arrive at the scene of an incident, they assess the patient's condition and take potentially life-saving decisions about any treatment needed before the patient is transferred to hospital. They use high-tech equipment, such as defibrillators (which restore the heart's rhythm), spinal and traction splints and intravenous drips, as well as administering oxygen and drugs. They then start giving the treatment, with the assistance of the ambulance technician.

Paramedics are trained to drive a mobile emergency clinic and to resuscitate and/or stabilise patients using techniques, equipment and drugs. They might be called out to a road traffic accident, or to someone with a heart attack. They work shifts, including evenings and weekends, going out in all weathers at all hours of the night or day. Often they work alongside other emergency services, such as the police or fire brigade. They may be based at a local ambulance station or a large hospital along with other emergency crews. They work closely with doctors and nurses in hospital accident and emergency departments, and also deal with patients' relatives and members of the public, some of whom may be upset and aggressive.

Paramedics may have had experience as an ambulance technician before becoming a paramedic. The direct entrant route is by qualifying at a university which offers courses approved by the Health Professions Council. Courses may be a diploma, foundation degree and/ or BSc honours degree in paramedic science. There are full-time courses for those applying through UCAS, and part time for those already working as qualified ambulance technicians. Courses last from two to five years, depending on whether they are full or part time. Entry requirements vary but a full, clean, manual driving licence of the appropriate class is also needed.

Research tip

Find out more from the British Paramedic Association at www.britishparamedic.org.

Medical laboratory technician

A medical laboratory technician is a clinical support worker. Clinical support workers and assistants work with doctors and scientists to diagnose and treat disease. They may work in pathology laboratories or work on wards or in clinics. In pathology laboratories, the clinical support worker's main role is as support to biomedical scientists. Their work involves a variety of laboratory skills such as: making up chemical solutions, using computers to analyse data, labelling and sorting of tissue samples, disposal of chemical or biological waste, maintaining stocks, and taking blood samples from patients.

Clinical support workers can work in biochemistry, histology, immunology, haematology, blood transfusion unit, and cytology. Clinical support workers may take blood (phlebotomy) or assist physiological scientists who are investigating the functioning of organ/body systems for example, ECG recordings.

Training is mostly on-the-job training, starting with an induction then specialised individual training such as NVQ level 2. This is a job where the skills escalator may be applicable.

Healthcare assistant

Healthcare assistants work in hospital or community settings under the guidance of a qualified healthcare professional, usually a nurse. They are sometimes known as auxiliary nurses. Healthcare assistants also work with qualified midwives in maternity services.

The work includes personal care for patients, such as washing and dressing, feeding, helping people to keep mobile, and taking them to the toilet, bedmaking and generally assisting patients. Sometimes the work includes taking temperatures, monitoring pulse, respirations. Nursing healthcare assistants usually work a 37.5-hour week on a shift or rota system, including nights and weekends. Many care assistants work part-time. Occasionally flexi-working is available.

Healthcare assistants may also work alongside healthcare scientists, for example helping audiologists with hearing tests. Clinical support workers (sometimes known as therapy assistants or therapy helpers) may work with allied health professionals such as physiotherapists, radiographers, podiatrists, speech and language therapists, dieticians and occupational therapists. Therapy assistants may prepare patients for their therapy, set up equipment, assist the therapist with the treatment and contribute to record keeping.

Key words

Histology – study of the structure of tissue
Haematology – study of blood and the body tissues which make it
Cytology – study of cells

Hospital play worker

Hospital play specialists use play as therapeutic tool. They work closely as part of the multi-disciplinary team, and organise daily play and art activities in the playroom or at the bedside, provide play to achieve developmental goals and help children cope with anxieties. Hospital play specialists may use play to prepare children for hospital procedures and to support families.

Children's hospitals have large play departments employing up to 40 hospital play specialists each. In general hospitals, small teams of play staff work in different areas of the hospital, such as out-patients clinics, children's units and adolescent wards.

Hospital play assistants need CACHE level 3 or NNEB (Nursery Nurses Examination Board) equivalent qualification or an NVQ Level 3 in Child Care. A hospital play specialist will need a Level 4 Diploma in Specialised Play for Sick Children and Young People. They may also need NHS training in child protection issues. The Edexcel Level 4 BTEC Professional Diploma in Specialised Play for Sick Children and Young People is required for application for professional registration with the hospital Play Staff Education Trust (HPSET). Both the qualification and professional registration together form the recognised National Health Service (NHS) qualification and standard for Hospital play staff. Play Staff Education Trust has applied to be registered with the Health Professions Council.

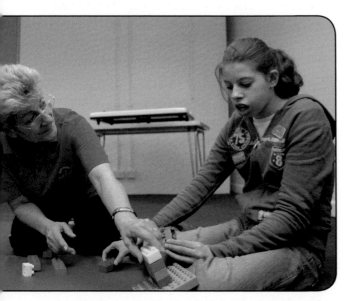

Figure 18.3 Specialists use play as a therapeutic tool

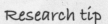

> ### Research tip
>
> Find out more about hospital play staff at www.hpset.org.uk.

Medical receptionist

A medical receptionist is usually the first person a patient or hospital visitor sees at reception when they visit a doctor, health centre or hospital. They welcome patients when they arrive, check details against the list of appointments that day, or record their details if the patient has arrived without an appointment. Increasingly the work involves the use of computers. Filing medical records and arranging future appointments for patients are important aspects of the job. Dealing with incoming mail and taking requests for repeat prescriptions, answering the telephone and recording requests for home visits are also part of the role.

Most medical receptionists work 37.5 hours a week which may include one or more evenings a week or they may have to work shifts. Some receptionists work in out-of-hours centres and hospitals so will have to work evenings, nights and at weekends. Part-time work may be available. Medical receptionists may have to deal with aggressive or anxious members of the public.

Training is given on the job. Some medical receptionists may study for qualifications offered by the Association of Medical Secretaries, Practice Managers, Administrators and Receptionists.

> ### Research tip
>
> Find out about the work of medical receptionists by looking at www.amspar.co.uk/.

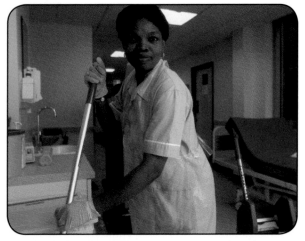

Figure 18.5 Domestic staff maintain cleanliness in hospitals

Domestic staff

Domestic staff are usually employed by an outside agency and contracted to work in different parts of a hospital. They maintain cleanliness in hospitals, cleaning the floors and emptying bins. Training is usually on the job. They may not work on the same wards each time but have to work on a variety of areas. They have to take great care when disposing of clinical waste so that they do not get injured. There are usually few entry requirements.

REQUIREMENTS

Competence

Competence means being skilled at something. You may be competent at making a bed, or organising your time. Both these competences will be useful in health care careers. Competences refer to skills – to things you can do.

Knowledge/Skills

Knowledge is something you know. You may know how important it is to a patient's comfort to have fresh sheets, but you may not be competent at bed-making. You may know how important it is to get to work on time, but not be competent at doing it.

Health careers at all levels require both knowledge

and competence. Medical students have to know normal blood values and be competent at taking blood. Midwives have to know what a normal position is for an unborn baby in the uterus and they have to be able to palpate the abdomen to recognise a normal position.

All careers require competence as well as knowledge and skills. Some careers require a great deal of knowledge; for example, doctors have to know how the body works (physiology), how it is structured (anatomy), how people interact (psychology) and how the chemicals in the body keep balance (biochemistry). Doctors must develop competences (skills); for example, a surgeon must develop competency with operative procedures.

Health and Social Care Apprenticeship – Health, Care and Public Services

The apprenticeship framework was originally developed for nursing but is now wider and includes health care careers, such as radiography. An apprentice working in health and social care helps senior care workers and social workers to provide care services.

The Skills Council for this sector is Skills for Health.

> ### Research tip
>
> Check out the website for Skills for Health: www.skillsforhealth.org.uk/.

Cadet schemes are planned to meet local needs. Trainees work in various parts of a hospital and are always supervised. They can see for themselves what careers are available. They may eventually go on to university and return as a qualified professional to the hospital where they once were a cadet.

Entry requirements for schemes vary. Some trusts do not ask for formal qualifications but ask for evidence of other skills, such as good time management and a caring attitude. Some trusts give successful trainees preferential status or an interview for a place on a pre-registration education programme at a local higher education institution. Information about what is available in your local area can be obtained from your local strategic health authority or local NHS trust(s).

Qualifications are not all the same. Some are purely vocational, such as National Vocational Qualifications. Some are a mixture of vocational and academic, for example, the BTEC qualifications. Some are purely academic, for example, A levels.

National Vocational Qualifications (NVQs)

NVQs are competence based. This means learners are assessed against a national set of standards. Learners are assessed on what they can do and either meet the standard or do not yet meet it. They can have another chance if they are not yet at the standard. People who are good at doing things rather than writing them down sometimes find NVQs suit them better. There are no age limits but carers must be 18 years old in order to perform personal care such as bathing people or helping them with toilet needs. NVQs are not fixed over a set period of time. Students can work at their own pace. An average time for an NVQ at level 3 may be 18 months but this varies with individual students. Work experience is essential for anyone taking an NVQ as they are assessed on what they can do in the workplace. An assessor observes the candidate doing their work and may ask the candidate why they did something. The candidate needs to know why a procedure is good practice as well as what is good practice. If the candidate meets the requirements they are said to be competent.

The role of the assessor is important in guiding and supporting the candidate at first so the candidate gets a clear idea of what they can do and what they need to improve on. The assessor helps the candidate to plan for assessment at a specific time, then becomes the judge of whether that candidate is competent.

There are different levels of NVQs:

- Level 1 requires an ability to perform routine activities. There is no level 1 in Care because people are unpredictable. A person who is happy one day may be aggressive or violent the

next and the worker must learn to work with a variety of situations.

- Level 2 requires workers to work under the direction of others.

- Level 3 requires workers to take more responsibility, supervising others. Carers who achieve level 3 NVQ may apply to university to do a nursing course.

- Level 4 is a managerial role requiring even more responsibility.

- Level 5 involves strategic planning and overall responsibility for an organisation.

BTECs

BTECs are work-related qualifications originally developed by the Business & Technology Education Council (BTEC). BTECs are offered as full-time courses from one to two years; short BTEC courses are also available. BTEC qualifications are recognised and available in over 50 countries.

Level 1 – BTEC Introductory

Level 1 qualifications give a broad introduction to a sector. They also provide a flavour of how BTECs work. An Introductory Certificate has four units: two core units, which everyone takes, a compulsory Personal Skills unit and one optional unit. The optional unit enables you to study an area in more depth. An Introductory Diploma has eight units: three core units, which everyone takes, two compulsory Personal Skills units and three optional units. The course is usually for one year.

Level 2 – BTEC First

Level 2 qualifications are good for those who have some GCSEs, but who want to do something different. They also develop skills and knowledge from Level 1. There is a certificate of three units: two core units, which everyone takes, and a choice of one specialist unit. The BTEC First certificate is equivalent to two GCSEs grades A*– C. The BTEC First Diploma is equivalent to four GCSEs grades A*– C. The Diploma is normally taken as a full-time course over one year. It contains six units: two core units that everyone takes and four specialist units.

Level 3 –BTEC National

These qualifications are at the same level as A levels but can get you a job as well as a university place. BTEC Nationals are well known and recognised by universities. They carry UCAS points. A BTEC National Diploma is based on national occupational standards and usually takes two years. Altogether 18 units are studied and there are three mandatory work placements. It is also possible to take a level 3 BTEC National Certificate with twelve units, and a BTEC National Award with six units. The BTEC National Award in Health and Social Care is planned as an additional qualification within a level 3 programme with GCEs.

The BTEC National Diploma (from Sept 2007) has the following pathways:

- Children's Care, Learning and Development

- Health and Social Care

- Health and Social Care (Health Sciences)

- Health and Social Care (Health Studies)

- Health and Social Care (Social Care).

The Health Sciences pathway provides the opportunity for more science-based units for those students wishing to enter health science careers. The health and social care pathway offers a balance of units for those students who have not yet decided on a final career choice in health and social care.

Level 4 – BTEC Higher National/BTEC Foundation Degree

These are BTEC's undergraduate qualifications roughly equivalent to the first half of a degree. A BTEC HND can get you onto the third year of many degree programmes but not into nursing or social work. Foundation degrees are planned for some professions allied to medicine.

Level 5 – BTEC Diploma in Management Studies

Level 5 qualifications are normally for managers wanting to gain more skills in a particular area. For example, the Diploma in Management Studies can take students onto an MBA at Heriot-Watt University.

A-Levels, GCE in Health and Social Care

A-levels give a broad understanding of the sector and some skills as well as technical knowledge and an awareness of particular groups and their needs by focusing on Health, Early Years (Care and Education), Care of Older People, or Individuals with Specific Needs. Unlike BTECs, these qualifications have some examined units. They do not have the workplace element so students take a theoretical approach to many subjects.

You can study for:

- Single Award AS GCE (3units): Units 1, 2, 3

- Double Award AS GCE (6 units): Units 1 to 6

- Single Award Advanced GCE (6 units): Units 1, 2, 3, 7, 8 and 9

- Double Award Advanced GCE (12 units): all units.

Specialised diploma

The specialised diploma has been developed for 14 to 19 year olds to provide a more vocational approach to learning than the A-level route. The specialist diploma Society, Health and Development covers the area of Care. There are three parts to the diploma: vocational or principal learning related to care; generic learning which includes English and maths as well as personal skills; and, finally, additional or specialist learning. The course includes practical activities such as visits, and a project which is internally assessed. The course includes ten days of work experience.

Levels of Diplomas - the Diploma is available at levels 1, 2 and 3:

- Level 1 Diploma will be comparable, in terms of average length of study, to a programme of four to five GCSEs

- Level 2 Diploma will be comparable, in terms of average length of study, to a programme of five to six GCSEs

- Level 3 Diploma will be comparable, in terms of average length of study, to a programme of three GCE A levels.

A level 3 award is also being developed, broadly comparable in size to two A levels.

Degrees

Degrees represent higher level study at level 4 or 5. Universities offer degrees on a full or part-time basis. Health care professions such as nursing, medicine and dentistry require a relevant degree and professional registration. It is possible to take a degree in health but not be a health care professional, and many people do take a degree in Health Studies or Health and Social Care out of general interest. Sometimes a relevant degree may help to fast track towards a professional degree if someone later decides they wish to become a health care professional.

The best way to find out what degrees are offered is to check the UCAS website (see below) and search for the degree you are interested in. You can search alphabetically by course, for example, searching for Physiotherapy brings up a list of universities which offer this degree. The University of Birmingham offers the three years full-time honours degree with state registration.

Research tip

You can find out more about degree courses by going to www.ucas.com. This site also gives information about entry requirements, how to apply, and funding arrangements.

Registration

Doctors, most nurses, midwives, dentists and occupational therapists all have to study to degree level in order to qualify. They must then register with the registering professional body. Sometimes, quite rarely, people study the degree then decide they do not want to be a doctor or nurse, and do not register with the professional body. They have the degree but cannot practise that profession until they register. The main professional bodies are listed below:

- The General Medical Council regulates the medical profession in the UK. Doctors must register with the GMC in order to practise.

- The General Dental Council registers and regulates the dental team.

- The Nursing and Midwifery Council registers all nurses and midwives and regulates the profession.

- The Health Professions Council registers health professions allied to medicine.

- The British Dietetic Association (BDA) is the professional association for dieticians.

- The British Association of Occupational Therapists (BAOT) is the professional body and trade union for occupational therapy staff in the UK. The College of Occupational Therapists is part of BAOT.

- The Royal Pharmaceutical Society of Great Britain (RPSGB) is the professional and regulatory body for pharmacists and pharmacy technicians in England, Scotland and Wales.

- The Chartered Society of Physiotherapy is the professional body for chartered physiotherapists, physiotherapy students and assistants.

- The professional body for paramedics is the British Paramedic Association.

Some jobs require no formal entry requirements; for example, medical receptionists, although employers are increasingly looking for candidates with GCSEs, or equivalent qualifications.

PERSONAL ATTRIBUTES

Anyone who works in health care should:

- have a friendly and sympathetic manner
- be calm, confident and well organised
- have strong team-working and communication skills
- be interested in working with people
- have a general interest in health issues.

Different careers require different knowledge but all jobs demand an ability to gain knowledge and skills in the relevant area. A radiographer must know about X-Rays. A nurse must know what a normal pulse rate is.

Interpersonal skills

In addition to subject knowledge, good *interpersonal skills* are essential in health care as we deal with members of the public, some of whom may be distressed. A person who has been waiting for hours to see a doctor may be in pain, angry and aggressive. Interpersonal skills – the skills for working with people – are essential to calm patients and relatives.

Initiative

Health care workers must be able to use their initiative, and should not wait to be told everything. If a drunken person comes into casualty on Saturday night and starts to throw chairs around, a health care worker should be able to use their initiative to call for assistance to manage the situation. *Confidence* is also needed when dealing with the public. A nurse who lacks confidence and is shy and hesitant will not inspire the patient with confidence. If the nurse seems unsure, the patient will begin to lose trust in the nurse and may panic.

Key words
initiative – doing something without being prompted by others

Empathy with others

Empathy with others is vital in health care. This is not sympathy, feeling sorry for someone in a sentimental way, but trying to put yourself in the patient's or relative's situation. A nurse who has empathy will understand that the aggressive relative swearing at staff in Casualty may be frightened, and the aggression reflects their fear of not being able to control events. They may need a firm but friendly approach and a clear explanation of what is happening.

Anti-discrimination approach

This is one of the most essential attributes of a health care worker. Personal prejudices must be shelved when on duty. You may not like people who drink and drive. You may think drug addicts bring it all on themselves. You may think everyone should learn English before they come to live in this country. But these are just your personal views and they must never affect your professional practice. Health care workers have a duty of care to all in need and cannot choose who to treat and who to turn away. This duty of care is part of what health care work is about. It is also a legal duty – enforceable by anti-discriminatory laws.

Ability to work with others

The ability to work with others is needed if a patient is to receive the best health care. There is no room for personal clashes in health care. You may not like everyone but you must be able to work with everyone. Just imagine what would happen in theatre if the scrub nurse did not want to work with the surgeon or the anaesthetist! The whole theatre list would be stopped while the nurse sulked. People might die. As a health care professional you have to work with everyone. If someone on the team does not pull their weight you have to work harder so that the patient does not suffer.

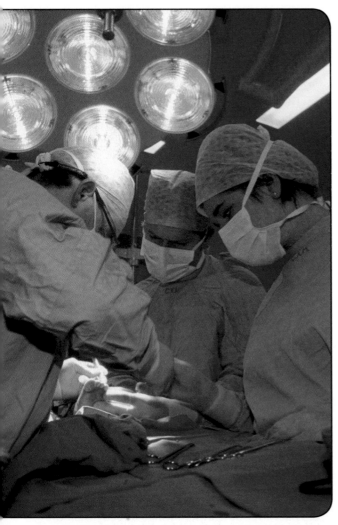

Figure 18.6 Good teamwork is essential in health care services

Reliability

Reliability is essential in health care. There is a lot of shift work, so a nurse may be on duty from 9pm to 8am the next morning. If you are unreliable and cannot arrive at work on time, that nurse will have to stay until you arrive. The same thing may happen to you when you are due to go off duty at 9pm. If the night nurse is unreliable and does not come in on time, you have to stay until the nurse arrives. It is important to say if you have not done something rather than hide it. A patient may be due to be discharged but needs to have stitches out first. If you are asked to remove the stitches and have been unable to do so, perhaps because you were dealing with another patient, you must say that you have not been able to do the job. Someone else on the team may then do it.

Ability to take responsibility for self and others

All health care professionals are responsible for their own performance, both for what they do and for what they do not do. A staff nurse may be dispensing medication. The nurse is responsible for giving the right medication to the right patient at the right time by the right route. The nurse must always check the patient's name and number. For example, there may be two Mary Smiths on the ward but the patient numbers will be different. The nurse must check if the medication is to be given orally or by another route such as by injection. The nurse is responsible for their own actions in giving medication. The nurse cannot delegate giving medication to an unqualified member of staff. The nurse is accountable for their own actions and for the actions of others if they inappropriately delegate a task to them. A receptionist must not be asked to give out medication. If the nurse does this and the wrong medicine is given, the nurse is responsible and risks being disciplined or losing their registration. Health care professionals are responsible for managing other staff and for managing the care of patients.

EVIDENCE ACTIVITY

P1, M1

P1 Describe the requirements for two careers in the health sector.

M1 Explain how the requirements of health care workers can contribute to providing a positive experience for patients.

You are thinking about a career in the health sector but are unsure what area to choose, so you decide to look at two careers to help you make up your mind. You need to explain to parents of potential students how these requirements can help patients. Write a brief report summarising your findings.

18.2 *Understand how organisations are structured in the health sector*

The health sector can appear confusing as there are many organisations offering different types of care.

The Department of Health sets national standards and shapes NHS and social care services, promoting healthier living in England. Health and social care services are delivered through the NHS, local authorities, arm's length bodies and other public and private sector organisations. The Department of Health is accountable to the public and the government for the overall performance of the NHS, personal social services and the work of the Department itself.

KEY ELEMENTS OF HEALTH AND SOCIAL CARE PROVISION

The key elements of health and social care provision can be seen in the diagram below.

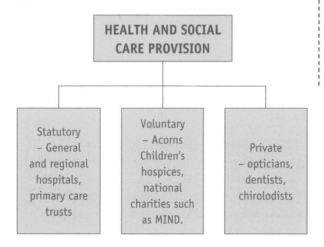

Figure 18.7 Organisation of health and social care provision

Statutory

Until 1990 most health and social care was provided by the state, i.e. it was statutory provision. Statutory, voluntary, private and informal providers of care became more equal partners in health and social care provision after the NHS and Community Care Act 1990.

Key words

Statutory – required by statute or written law; a state requirement

Statutory provision for health care in a community would include a large general hospital and the local GP service.

Voluntary

Voluntary provision includes national and local charities. National charities, such as MIND, provide advice and support for people with mental health issues in England and Wales. A local charity may fund a hospice in a local area for those with a terminal illness.

Example

Acorns children's hospices are local charities which offer care in the West Midlands to life-limited children and their families 24 hours a day, seven days a week.

Acorns get over 80% of its income directly from the public. Less than 20% of their funding comes from government sources.

Research tip

Find out more about Acorns hospices. Go to www.acorns.org.uk

Private provision

Private provision is paid for directly by the patient at the time. Opticians charge for eye tests and for spectacles. Many dentists now charge for treatment and offer only private provision. People needing an operation may choose to have it done in the private sector, for example at a BUPA hospital.

CASE STUDY: PRIVATE HEALTHCARE

Neetha has very bad toothache and goes to see her NHS dentist. He tells her her wisdom teeth are impacted and all 4 will need to be removed in hospital under anaesthetic. The waiting time for a consultation with the hospital dentist is 3 months and the wait for surgery is a further 6 months. Neetha is in a lot of pain and can't wait that long. Fortunately for her she is covered for dental treatment by her company medical insurance and is able to go private. She sees the hospital dentist the next day and has her wisdom teeth removed 1 day later.

QUESTION

What objections could some people have to the use of private provision?

Social services

Social services are services provided by the government at a local level. Health is administered nationally, but social services are administered by your local authority. The Children Act 2004 requires all local authorities to create new accountabilities for children's services. In some areas, social services are now organised under the directorate of Adults and Communities and the directorate of Children, Young People and Families.

Social care services look after the health and welfare of the population. Some of the main groups using the services include children or families who are under stress, people with disabilities, people with emotional or psychological difficulties, people with financial or housing problems and older people who need help with daily living activities.

Social care services may be offered in hospitals or health centres, in educational settings, in community groups, in residential homes, advice centres or even in people's own homes. Social care services are normally run by local councils, sometimes in conjunction with local NHS providers and organisations. Many councils work together to run social care services.

The Commission for Social Care Inspection inspects and regulates all social care providers in England and publishes reports on the performance of local councils in delivering social care. The Commission's website allows the public to search the directory of care homes and other services in England; and obtain free copies of inspection reports about each care home or service.

Research tip

Check out some care homes in your area by going to the CSCI website www.csci.org.uk

National Health Service (NHS)

The National Health Service is responsible for all health services in England and Wales. Strategic Health Authorities (SHAs) manage the NHS locally and are a key link between the Department of Health and the NHS.

Strategic health authorities (SHAs)

England is split into 10 strategic health authorities (SHAs). One of the functions of SHAs is to commission places for nursing from local universities. The SHA tells the nursing departments how many nurses they need, and the university then offers that number of places.

SHAs develop plans for improving health services in their local area and make sure their local NHS organisations perform well. Within each SHA, the NHS is split into various types of trusts that take responsibility for running the different NHS services in the local area. SHAs are also responsible for making sure national priorities are integrated into local health service plans so, for example, national programmes for improving cancer services are linked to local provision.

There are several different types of trust, outlined below.

Acute trusts

Acute trusts make sure that hospitals provide high-quality healthcare, and spend their money efficiently. Acute trusts decide how each hospital will develop and improve services. These acute trusts employ nurses, doctors, pharmacists, midwives and health visitors, physiotherapists, radiographers, podiatrists, speech and language therapists, counsellors, occupational therapists and psychologists. They also employ non-medical staff such as receptionists, porters, cleaners, specialists in information technology, and domestic and security staff.

Increasingly some acute trusts are becoming regional specialist centres. Local hospitals are losing specialist facilities which then go to the regional centre. Regional centres are often linked to universities and become training centres for the nurses and doctors of the future.

Foundation trusts

NHS Foundation Trusts ('foundation hospitals') are a new type of NHS Trust in England. They have power to make decisions on strategy and finance and are more responsive to local needs. Foundation trusts are run by local managers, staff and representatives of the public. They offer services according to the needs of the area, so if there is a high incidence of kidney problems in an area for example, they may develop a specialist renal unit. NHS Foundation Trusts represent a profound change in way in which hospital services are managed. Previously they were managed centrally; now they are being managed locally.

Ambulance trusts

Ambulance trusts provide emergency care such as rapid response teams. In some areas they also provide some transport for patients to get to hospital.

Care trusts

Care trusts work in both health and social care. They carry out a range of services, including social care, mental health services or primary care services. Care trusts are set up when the NHS and local authorities agree to work together, usually where it is felt that a closer relationship between health and social care is needed or would benefit local care services.

Mental health trusts

Mental health trusts provide care for people with mental health problems. They offer counselling in the community and community psychiatric nursing as well as more acute care.

Primary care trusts

Primary care trusts provide the first care. This care may be provided by the the local doctor (GP) or the NHS dentist. Primary care trusts also provide NHS walk-in centres and NHS Direct telephone help. The government puts most of the money for health care into primary care trusts so that local services provide care to meet local needs.

Special health authorities

These include the National Blood Authority, which serves the whole of the country.

Secondary health care

Secondary health care relates to the second type of health care you may receive after you have seen your GP or optician or dentist. It includes hospital and day centre care.

Booked admissions will give patients a choice of appointments and admission dates, speeding up the service for patients. Some hospitals have had to be reorganised to enhance the range of secondary services available locally. Accident and emergency facilities are now centralised at major hospitals where full teams provide a service 24 hours a day. There has been an increase in day surgery and reduced hospital stays for many operations. Some treatments such as minor surgery and diagnostic procedures are now offered at treatment centres.

Some health care is now delivered for the NHS by the private sector. Private hospitals are paid by the NHS to perform investigations and minor surgery to reduce waiting list times. Support workers have been brought in to help radiographers with screening programmes and the use of support workers is being extended in professions allied to medicine.

Integrated care

Care trusts (see page 146), which were introduced in 2002, are a combination of current NHS and local authority services. Care trusts provide improved customer-focused services which are responsive to local needs. However, in caring for people with learning disabilities, the medical model of care is not always appropriate.

People with learning disabilities now have Learning Disability Partnership Boards and the Valuing People support team as well as the learning Disability Task Force to represent their views. The National Forum for People with Learning Difficulties can influence what happens locally.

The social model of disability is more appropriate for people with learning disabilities. This client group may be disadvantaged by a medical model of care. The Department of Health suggests that care trusts must use a person-centred approach and involve people with learning disabilities as equal partners in decisions which affect them. Partnership with local authorities, Connexions and the other partnerships formed to deliver LD services locally must be maintained.

Integrated care opportunities arise in planning continuing care, tackling delayed hospital discharges or transfers, and pooling money and other resources. The Health Act 1999 allows and encourages resources and management structures to be integrated.

Children's trusts

Children's trusts bring together all the professionals involved with children so they can work together for the benefit of children in their care. The aim is to break down professional barriers, reduce duplication and improve service. The Common Assessment Framework is used to share information and plan care together so that schools, social workers, doctors and community nurses are all aware of what is being done to help a child.

Accountability for meeting statutory duties is retained but services may be provided differently. Listening to the views of children and young people is an important aspect of children's trusts.

This is commonly referred to as the DFES model. See Unit 17 page 114 for an example.

HEALTH SETTINGS

Traditional health settings are changing as government policy demands a more responsive service and shorter waiting lists. Long-stay hospital wards are closing and more day care units are being opened. There is a trend to admit fewer people to hospital, dealing with cases of minor surgery in primary care settings such as health centres. Only those who are acutely ill stay in hospital. Children are no longer kept in hospital for long periods but are cared for at home. Patients with cancer are admitted for a few hours of chemotherapy and recover at home.

More primary care in the community means that patients with mental health issues will be cared for at home, with the support of a community psychiatric nurse. Older people now have a choice of remaining at home and having care at home rather than being admitted to residential care.

> ***Think*** What are the potential problems of treating mental health issues in the community?

More care is carried out in the community – in primary care centres and at home. GPs must now meet performance targets and manage their practice financially as well as offering more services. Some offer counselling, smoking cessation and health promotion advice. The expansion of primary care is set to continue as PCTs are the biggest employers of NHS staff and have 80% of the NHS budget.

ACCESS TO HEALTH SERVICES

Health services may be available locally but there are still people who, for different reasons, do not or cannot use these services.

Barriers to access

Barriers to access may be because of specific needs. A person who is terminally ill with cancer may be too depressed or feel unable to travel 30 miles to a regional centre for chemotherapy. An illegal immigrant may be reluctant to visit a GP for a chest infection because they are scared of being arrested and deported.

Financial reasons may prevent people accessing services. Older people and others who have limited means may struggle to find the bus fare to attend an outpatient's appointment. The drugs they need may not be provided by the local PCT as it may have been deemed too expensive. Herceptin is one drug which was not freely available until public pressure caused a rethink on the matter. The National Institute for Health and Clinical Excellence (NICE) monitors the effectiveness of drugs and advises what is cost effective.

There may be geographical barriers which prevent access to services. Homeless people cannot get access to a GP because they have no home address. There is also a 'postcode lottery' effect where one PCT may allow GPs to prescribe a treatment, whereas another PCT does not fund that treatment. For example, In Vitro Fertilisation (IVF) treatment is subject to such variation.

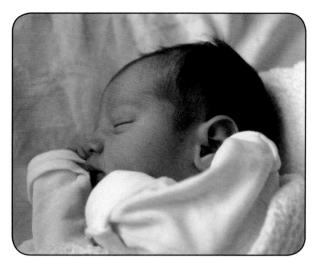

Figure 18.8 IVF treatment may not be available on the NHS in all areas

There may be social barriers which prevent people accessing services. Medical receptionists may be unwelcoming to new patients. GPs have a right to refuse to take patients on their list. Some GPs can be reluctant to take drug addicts or smokers on their list, for example, as they will cost the practice a lot of money in managing their addiction. Socially the GP may feel that they have brought the problems on themselves.

There can be cultural reasons why people do not access services. For example, someone might be reluctant to admit that they suspect they have a sexually transmitted disease. They may be intimidated by an abusive partner or reluctant to ask for help in coping with a partner's alcoholism. They may come from a culture where it is not acceptable to be sick, especially if they have a highly pressured job and are continually under a lot of stress.

NATIONAL SERVICE FRAMEWORKS

The New NHS and *Saving Lives: Our Healthier Nation* set out measures intended to improve the quality of services to patients, and to reduce variations in health and the provision of services. These White Papers, together with the tobacco White Paper *Smoking Kills*, introduced NSFs to improve health, reduce inequalities and raise the quality of care. National Service Frameworks (NSFs) are long-term strategies for improving specific areas of care. They set measurable goals within set time frames.

Coronary heart disease

The NSF for coronary heart disease (CHD) was launched in 2000 and sets 12 standards for improved prevention, diagnosis and treatment, and goals to secure fair access to high quality services. The standards are to be implemented over a 10-year period.

CHD is common, frequently fatal, and largely preventable. It kills more than 110,000 people a year in England. More than 1.4 million people in the UK suffer from angina and about 300,000 people have a heart attack each year. Unskilled working men are three times more likely to die prematurely of CHD than men in professional or managerial occupations. The wives of manual workers have nearly twice the risk compared to the wives of non-manual workers. Angina, heart attack and stroke are all more common amongst those in manual social classes.

For people born in the Indian sub-continent, the death rate from heart disease is 38% higher for men and 43% higher for women than rates for the country as a whole. Services for CHD vary regionally and the death rate from CHD in people under 65 is almost three times higher in Manchester than in Richmond. Areas with less CHD have better services.

Standards include reducing heart disease and preventing CHD in high-risk patients. They set targets for GPs and primary health care teams to identify all people at significant risk of cardiovascular disease but who have not developed symptoms and offer them appropriate advice and treatment to reduce their risks. One of the targets is that people with symptoms of a possible heart attack should receive help from an individual equipped with and appropriately trained in the use of a defibrillator within 8 minutes of calling for help. People thought to be suffering from a heart attack should be assessed professionally and, if indicated, receive aspirin. Thrombolysis (clot busting drugs) should be given within 60 minutes of calling for professional help. Cardiac rehabilitation is one of the targets set to reduce the risk of subsequent cardiac problems.

Cancer

The NHS Cancer Plan (2000) addresses health inequalities through setting targets for the reduction of smoking rates and promoting a healthier diet. Raising awareness and increasing screening are actions to reduce cancer rates.

Waiting times are to be reduced and investment in specialist palliative care increased by training more nurses in palliative care and by linking with the Macmillan Nursing service, which trains cancer nurse specialists. The cancer workforce, cancer facilities, and cancer research are to be expanded.

Paediatric intensive care

The National Service Framework for paediatric intensive care was established in 1999.

It calls for more post-registration students and training in advanced life support, and recommends a flexible approach to education. Paediatric intensive care facilities are to be expanded to meet needs.

Mental health

The NSF for mental health was launched in 1999. The NSF lists seven standards that set targets for the mental health care of adults aged up to 65. Care of those over 65 is included in the NSF for older people. These standards span five areas: health promotion and stigma, primary care and access to specialist services, needs of those with severe and enduring mental illness, carers' needs, and suicide reduction.

Older people

The NSF for older people launched in 2001 sets national standards for care across health and social services for all older people whether they live at home, in residential care or are being cared for in hospital.

Diabetes

This NSF was launched in 1999 and aims to help the 1.3 million people with diabetes in England. Standards aim to provide good care and reduce inequality of provision. Target areas include: preventing and identifying diabetes; empowering people with diabetes; clinical care for adults, children and young people with diabetes; managing diabetic emergencies and care of people with diabetes in hospital; diabetes and pregnancy and detection and management of long-term complications.

Long-term conditions

The NSF for long-term conditions was published in 2005. The aim is to improve the lives of the 15 million people who live with neurological and other long-term conditions by providing them with better health and social care services. Long-term conditions are those conditions that cannot, at present, be cured, but can be controlled by medication and other therapies.

Key themes are independent living, person-centred care, easier access to services and joint working across all agencies and disciplines involved, such as providers of transport, housing, employment, education, benefits and pensions.

This NSF is a way of delivering support for people with long-term conditions outlined in the White Paper *Our Health, Our Care, Our Say* and the NHS Improvement Plan: *Putting People at the Heart of Public Services*.

The long-term (neurological) conditions NSF has similar targets around person-centred care planning, information and support, self-care and case management.

Renal

The NSF for renal services is in two parts. Part one sets five standards which will help the NHS and its partners manage demand, increase fairness of access and improve choice and quality in dialysis and kidney transplant services. Part two sets four quality requirements and identifies good practice to help limit the development and progression of chronic kidney disease; minimise the impact of acute renal failure; and extend palliative care to people dying with kidney failure.

Children

This NSF, published in 2004, sets standards for children's health, social services, and the interface of those services with education. Health visitors' roles are increasingly under pressure and there is a lack of consistency in the services offered to families and a lack of clarity about the role of health visitors. The Children's NSF is intended to result in services being designed and delivered around the needs of children and families. The Children's NSF is aimed at everyone who comes into contact with, or delivers services to children, young people or pregnant women. The standards listed below focus on providing support, early intervention and joint working.

1 Promoting Health and Well-being, Identifying Needs and Intervening Early

2 Supporting Parenting

3 Child, Young Person and Family-Centred Services

4 Growing up into Adulthood

5 Safeguarding and Promoting the Welfare of Children and Young People

6 Children and Young People who are Ill

7 Children and Young People in Hospital

8 Disabled Children and Young People and Those with Complex Health Needs

9 The Mental Health and Psychological Well-being of Children and Young People

10 Medicines for Children and Young People

11 Maternity Services.

Patient-centred practice

Patient-centred practice is at the heart of all the NSFs, in an effort to improve the health of the nation and change the culture of the NHS from being task centred to a patient-centred approach. Reducing inequalities in health, empowering people to make healthy choices and enabling them to maintain a healthy lifestyle are values underpinning the NSFs.

CHILDREN AND YOUNG PEOPLE

Every Child Matters (2003) was the government response to the death of Victoria Climbié (see page 122, Unit 17). It focused on the care of children and young people from birth to age 19. The government's aim is for every child to have the support they need to:

- Be healthy

- Stay safe

- Enjoy and achieve

- Make a positive contribution

- Achieve economic well-being.

Joint working between hospitals, schools, police and voluntary groups will ensure sharing of information to protect children and young people from harm. Children and young people should have a voice in what happens to them. Integrated services, children's trusts, consisting of local authorities and partners will work together and involve children when planning. A Children's Commissioner for England was appointed in 2005, to give children and young people a voice.

The Children's Fund identifies children and young people at risk of social exclusion, and makes sure they receive the support they need.

A Common Assessment Framework (CAF) provides a national, common process for early assessment to identify all the child's individual, family and community needs, which can be built up over time and shared between practitioners. A common process reduces duplication and streamlines assessment.

Extended schooling is a way of delivering the outcomes for *Every Child Matters* and aims to improve attendance and achievement. An extended school works with local providers, agencies (and other schools) to provide a core of integrated services:

- wraparound childcare all year round (in primary schools)

- parenting and family support

- activities including study support, sport and music clubs

- easy referral to specialist services such as health and social care

- community use of facilities, including adult and family learning and ICT.

England, Wales, Northern Ireland and Scotland vary in their provision of care.

EVIDENCE ACTIVITY

P2

P2 Describe the overall structure of health services provision in home country.

You are the public relations officer for a foundation trust hospital and need to describe the overall structure of health service provision in your area to introduce an item for the Trust news letter. You may use labelled diagrams to help you explain the overall structure.

18.3 Understand roles and responsibilities in the health sector

OVERARCHING ORGANISATIONS

Roles and responsibilities

The Department of Health has overall responsibility for health and social care in England. This is delivered by the NHS and social services. At a national level the Department works with strategic health authorities (SHAs) and arm's length bodies (ALBs).

Skills for Health is the Sector Skills Council (SSC) for the UK health sector. It helps to deliver a skilled and flexible UK workforce in order to improve health and healthcare.

The National Institute for Health and Clinical Excellence (NICE) is an independent organisation responsible for providing national guidance on the promotion of good health and the prevention and treatment of ill health. NICE produces guidance on public health, health technologies and on clinical practice.

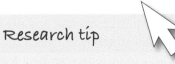

Research tip

Find out more about NICE and the work they do go to www.nice.org.uk/

The Health Protection Agency (HPA) is an independent body that protects the health and well-being of the population. The Agency helps protect people from infectious diseases and prevents harm when hazards involving chemicals, poisons or radiation occur. They also prepare for threats, such as a bio-terrorist attack or virulent new strain of disease.

Public Health Observatories are a network of 12 public health observatories (PHOs) working across England, Scotland, Wales, Northern Ireland and the Republic of Ireland and linking with those in Europe and beyond. The Association (APHO) facilitates joint working to turn raw data into meaningful health intelligence.

ROLE OF WORKFORCE DEVELOPMENT

Strategic Health Authorities (SHAs) work with the Workforce Development Confederations (WDCs) to co-ordinate the action needed to develop the NHS workforce. They encourage approaches that help people to achieve their full potential; optimise individual and team contributions to individually focused care; facilitate flexibility in workforce planning; and support the extension of existing roles and the development of new roles.

WDCs work to increase transferability of competence and qualifications; they try to ensure that managers and deliverers of healthcare receive education and training that equips them with the competences needed to safely undertake their work. Continuing professional development and continuing professional competence are part of a professional health care worker's role. In periods of transition, where roles are continually changing and succession planning is needed, it is essential for staff always to be up to date.

National occupational standards set out the competences for areas of work. Agenda for Change is more than a pay system. It allows employers to design jobs around the needs of patients, define the core skills and knowledge they want staff to develop in each job and pay extra when they face staffing difficulties. The skills escalator mentioned at the beginning of the unit (page 131) will be relevant here. The NHS Knowledge and Skills Framework supports personal and career progression. This is linked to annual development reviews and monitoring of personal development plans.

EVIDENCE ACTIVITY

P3, M2

P3 Describe the roles and responsibilities of three overarching organisations in the health sector.

M2 Explain the roles of the three organisations in improving health services provision.

As press officer for the hospital trust you want the newsletter to be distributed a week before the next public meeting. You wish to inform readers about three overarching organisations in the health sector but you have to assume your audience knows little about the organisations, their roles or responsibilities.

Therefore your article needs to describe clearly the roles and responsibilities of three overarching organisations in the health sector. Your audience will appreciate diagrams or pictures to support your description. 'Overarching' means 'being part of the big picture' so you will need three large providers. 'Roles' are what the organisations do. Responsibilities include who they are responsible to. You may like to use a table to help your audience understand each section:

	Roles	Responsible to
Organisation 1		
Organisation 2		
Organisation 3		

You anticipate some opposition at the public meeting and want to show the public how these organisations have improved health care provision, so you draft a leaflet to be handed to each person as they arrive. The leaflet will need an eye-catching title and should explain the roles of the three organisations in improving health services provision.

LEGISLATION AND GUIDANCE

Legislation relevant to this area includes:

- The National Health Service Act 2006;
- The National Health Service (Wales) Act 2006;
- The National Health Service (Consequential Provisions) Act 2006.

The National Health Service Act sets out the roles for Strategic Health Authorities, Primary Care Trusts, NHS Trusts, and Special Health Authorities.

The Health and Social Care (Community Health and Standards) Act 2003 created the Commission for Social Care Inspection (CSCI), a single, independent inspectorate for all social care services in England. National minimum standards are guidelines set out by the Department of Health as important guidelines to help providers, inspectors and people who use services to judge the standard of service.

Organisational policies and procedures are drawn from key legislation, charters and codes of practice. As well as covering legal requirements for anti-discriminatory practice and health and safety, policies will govern joint working arrangements in the changing world of health care.

ACCOUNTABILITIES AND REDRESS

Accountabilities to professional bodies have already been mentioned but there is also accountability to the line manager when employed. At times there may be conflict, for example if a manager asks a nurse or doctor to work when staffing levels are inadequate. The first duty of care is to the patient and the professional must always remember that they alone are accountable for their work. A disciplinary hearing will not accept the plea that 'a manager told me to do it'. Professionals are accountable for their own practice.

There are procedures for complaints both internally and externally. Trade unions usually have local representatives who will accompany members to hearings. In some cases, professional associations are the regulatory bodies and may conduct their own hearings in a case of alleged misconduct. 'Whistle blowing', or reporting of bad practice, is a last resort to be used if all else fails. It must be done sensitively to protect patients.

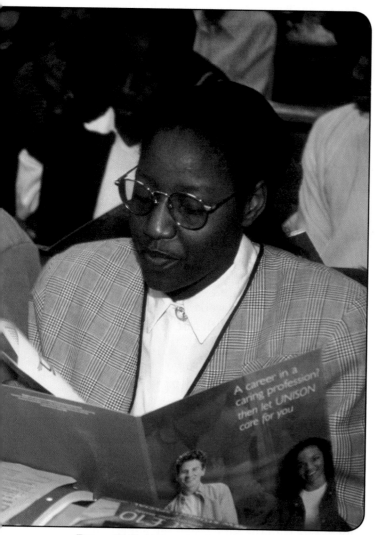

Figure 18.9 *Unison is the trade union representing people delivering public services*

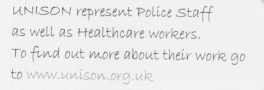

Research tip

UNISON represent Police Staff as well as Healthcare workers. To find out more about their work go to www.unison.org.uk

EVIDENCE ACTIVITY

P4, M3

P4 Describe three examples of legislation, policies, standards or codes of practice that influence provision of health services.

M3 Explain the role of legislation, policies, standards or codes of practice in improving provision of health services.

Prepare an induction pack for new staff at the hospital trust to show three examples of how legislation, policies, standards or codes of practice influence provision of health services. You will need to explain in the pack how each example has improved the provision of health services. New staff may be from any job role in the Trust so the pack must be easily understood by all.

EVIDENCE ACTIVITY

P5, D1

P5 Explain the role of workforce development in the health sector.

D1 Evaluate the requirements of health care workers in terms of providing a competent workforce for the health sector.

Part of your role involves working in the human resources department. Your boss asks you to prepare a presentation to explain the role of workforce development in the health sector and to evaluate the requirements of health care workers in terms of providing a competent workforce for the health sector.

18.4 *Understand multi-disciplinary working in the health sector*

EXAMPLES OF WORKING IN PARTNERSHIP

Examples may be seen in Children's Trusts, where multi-agency working puts the service users at the heart of planning and decision making.

The national service framework for long-term conditions involves primary care trusts liaising with NHS trusts, social services and charitable organisations.

Local university departments work in partnership with SHAs and hospital trusts to plan training of staff for the health service.

PURPOSE OF WORKING IN PARTNERSHIP

A holistic approach benefits patients. Partners identify common aims and objectives with the client. This approach promotes integration, reduces duplication, maximises resources and ensures a consistent approach which is especially important where clients are vulnerable. Working in partnership benefits the NHS as a more efficient skill mix of staff may be allocated to provide the best possible care at the least cost to the tax payer.

EVIDENCE ACTIVITY

P6, M4, D2

P6 Describe two examples of multi-disciplinary working in the health sector.

M4 Explain how multi-disciplinary working can improve the provision of health services.

D2 Use examples to evaluate the effectiveness of multi-disciplinary working for patients.

You are hoping for an early night but a colleague goes off sick and you are asked to step in to explain multi-disciplinary working in the health sector to the Trust governors tomorrow. You need to prepare a talk which lasts for about five minutes and you will need to provide notes so your colleague knows what you said in their absence.

The talk must describe two examples of multi-disciplinary working in the health sector and explain how it can improve the provision of health services. You should also use examples to evaluate the effectiveness of multi-disciplinary working for patients.

Health Education

unit 20

In this unit you will examine the principles and approaches used to educate people about health and well being. You will look at various types of health education campaigns as well as gaining an understanding of the historical, national and international influences on health. As an aspect of health promotion, this unit links to public health issues which are explored in greater depth in Unit 12: Public Health.

You will develop your knowledge and understanding of how people are influenced to change their attitudes and behaviours towards health. Different approaches to health education will be examined, including the role of the mass media and social marketing.

This unit will provide you with the information that you need to carry out your own health education campaign. This will be a small-scale activity requiring you to plan, design, implement and evaluate a campaign on a health related topic of your own choice. This will form the basis for a major part of the assessment for this unit.

Learning outcomes

On completion of this unit you will:

So, you want to be a...

Health promotion worker

My name Andy Ivamy
Age 26
Income £25,000

If you are passionate about promoting a healthy lifestyle this varied and exciting job could be for you.

What do you do?

Currently I am managing a project on breakfast clubs. I started by identifying schools and helping them to apply for funding. I also provided practical advice about how to go about setting up the breakfast club. I train those who run the clubs and generally promote healthy eating throughout the schools and in the curriculum. Jamie Oliver's programme on TV gave my job quite a boost.

What are your responsibilities?

I manage the projects, which includes monitoring and evaluating the clubs to see that they are meeting their targets. I give training to the workers and often provide practical demonstrations of healthy eating to school staff, parents and children. I do presentations to head teachers and other organisations. I have to be aware of how my work fits in with the government's guidelines on healthy eating for schools.

How did you get your job?

When I first left university I was lucky to get a job with my local primary care trust co-ordinating their exercise programme for people who had suffered heart attacks. I had undertaken some work experience with the health promotion department when I was at university so I heard about the job and was able to apply when it was advertised.

What training did you get?

While I was at college I really enjoyed studying a variety of health-related subjects such as health promotion, health studies, public health, nutrition, dietetics, environmental health, social science, community and youth work. I then studied for a degree in psychology. My work experience working in different health care settings has been invaluable and helped me to get my first job. I now get on-going training as part of my job.

> **"We sometimes do some health promotion activities in pubs and nightclubs"**

What are the hours like?

It all depends what I am doing! Obviously breakfast clubs can mean an early start. We sometimes do some health promotion activities in interesting places like pubs and nightclubs. On the whole the hours are varied.

What skills do you need?

You need an interest in health improvement and a broad understanding of the determinants of health. As you meet so many different people you need to be good at building and maintaining relationships with different individuals and organisations. As in many jobs you need good communication skills; the ability to make decisions, manage your time and solve problems.

Grading criteria

The table shows what you need to do to gain a pass, merit or distinction in this part of the qualification. Make sure you refer back to it when you are completing work so you can judge whether you are meeting the criteria and what you need to do to fill in gaps in your knowledge or experience.

In this unit there are three evidence activities that give you an opportunity to demonstrate your achievement of the grading criteria

page 170	P1 and M1
page 174	P2
page 185	P3, P4, P5, M2, M3, M4, D1 and D2

To achieve a pass grade the evidence must show that the learner is able to...	To achieve a merit grade the evidence must show that, in addition to the pass criteria, the learner is able to...	To achieve a distinction grade the evidence must show that, in addition to the pass and merit criteria, the learner is able to...
P1 Explain three different approaches to health education	**M1** Compare three different approaches to health education	
P2 Describe two different models of behaviour change, and the importance of the social and economic context		
P3 Describe the design and implementation of own small scale health education campaign	**M2** Explain the approaches and methods used in own health education campaign, relating them to models of behaviour change	**D1** Evaluate the approaches and methods used in own health education campaign, relating them to models of behaviour change
P4 Explain how own health education campaign met the aims and objectives, and explain the ethical issues involved	**M3** Analyse how own health education campaign met the aims and objectives and addressed any ethical issues	
P5 Explain how own small scale health education campaign links to local/national/international targets and strategies for health.	**M4** Analyse the role of own small scale health education campaign in terms of local/national/international targets and strategies for health.	**D2** Evaluate own health education campaign.

20.1 *Understand different approaches to health education*

Health as a concept means different things to different people. The World Health Organization defined health like this:

Health is a state of complete physical, mental, and social well being, not merely the absence of disease and infirmity. (WHO 1946)

Unit 7 looked at different concepts of health and ill health, including the biomedical and socio-medical models of health. By identifying which aspect of health is the most important, the appropriate model of health education can be used as the basis to make changes in attitudes and behaviours. The most common approaches are:

- medical or preventive
- behaviour change
- educational
- empowerment
- social change.

Key words

Empowerment – increasing the political, social or economic strength of an individual or community by increasing skills and confidence.

CASE STUDY: MR JONES

Mr Jones is 87 years old and lives alone since his wife died 3 years ago. He has arthritis and a bad hip, and finds it difficult to walk any distance. His flat is on the top floor and has poor heating. He gets very lonely at times. His wife did most of the cooking and he is finding it hard to eat well. His diet mainly consists of tinned food as he does not get to the shops to get fresh food very regularly. He has started to neglect himself as he finds it too much of an effort to get bathed and to do his washing. He used to belong to some local clubs, in particular the Old Comrades. They served together in the forces and now meet up to share their memories and enjoy a drink in the pub. He has not attended the meetings for a while and feels that his presence has not been missed. His family are very concerned about him and have contacted various agencies to try to improve the situation. They have been interested in the different approaches that different professionals have taken. His doctor is keen that Mr Jones should have an operation on his hip as he feels that if his physical health problems are overcome he will get back to his old self. The care manager wants to help him to change some of his unhealthy habits. She would like him to eat better and to care for himself. She is trying to get him to attend a day care centre regularly where he will meet people and have nourishing meals. At the day centre they also have talks about health and healthy eating for older people and an opportunity to practise cooking. Mr Jones' grand-daughter has recently visited him and discussed with him what he would like to happen. She was interested to learn that his choices for the future were different from what she had expected. He would like to go into a nearby residential home which is especially for people who have served in the armed forces. The family had always thought he would not want to leave his flat. She set about making enquiries and the family was amazed to find how, once a place was identified for him in the home he had chosen, he took on a new lease of life. He is now busy planning his move.

QUESTIONS

1. What approaches did the professionals such as the social worker and doctor take to improving the health of Mr Jones?

2. What approach did the family and Mr Jones himself take?

HISTORICAL PERSPECTIVE

Development of public health system

Two thousand years ago the Romans understood the importance of public health and you can still see the public baths that they built in the town of Bath. There was an understanding of the importance of hygiene to good health.

However it was during the nineteenth century that the main foundations of today's public health systems were laid and health campaigns took place. Two individuals stand out in the fight against disease caused by the unsanitary conditions in which many people lived: Edwin Chadwick and Dr John Snow (see page 78). A series of reforms to improve the physical environment such as the water supply, poor housing, the disposal of rubbish and sewage led to this being called the 'golden age' of public health.

There were also other developments which contributed to the general improvement in health of the population. Doctors and other researchers began to understand more about the causes and the origins of many diseases. For example, an English doctor called Edward Jenner produced a vaccine against smallpox in 1796. Health education campaigns led to the eventual elimination of smallpox worldwide, declared by the WHO in 1977. Gradually the importance of health education became more recognised. From early exhortations to take the 'sea air' in Victorian times, more sophisticated messages were developed. Doctors, nurses, health visitors and others gave advice on how to stay healthy by eating well and taking fresh air and exercise.

Health campaigns were targeted at certain issues, such as sexually transmitted diseases or alcohol misuse. Many poor people drank gin during the eighteenth century. It was cheap and seen as a quick escape from the terrible working and living conditions experienced by the poor. Women drank it as well as men and it became known as 'Mother's ruin'. Eventually during the nineteenth century there was concerted action against the perils and dangers of alcohol, with the rise of the temperance movement set up to educate and change people's behaviour by encouraging sobriety and total abstinence.

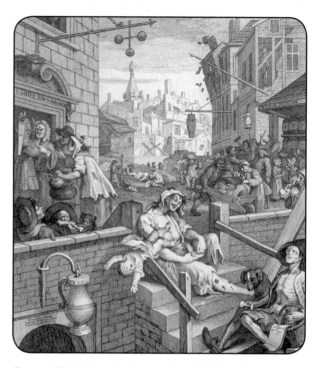

Figure 20.1 Hogarth's painting Gin Lane portrays the poor as drunk and degenerate

The twentieth century saw a more sophisticated understanding of the biological causes of diseases. Health became defined by the medical model which sees health as the absence of disease and encourages a scientific or medical solution. Preventative measures, such as immunisation and screening leading to the early detection of diseases, have been used to improve the health of individuals. In 1942 the Beveridge Report was commissioned by the government as part of the effort to rebuild Britain after the Second World War. It recommended that action should be taken to counteract the five 'giant evils' of 'Want, Disease, Ignorance, Squalor and Idleness.' This was the basis of the Welfare State which resulted in the founding of the National Health Service in 1948. It was to provide healthcare for all citizens, based on need – not the ability to pay. Health education continued to be based on the control of infectious diseases and accident prevention. In the 1950s the British Medical Association (BMA) launched a magazine called *Family Doctor* which included articles about the promotion of health and prevention of disease. Gradually it became apparent that the idealistic view that a National

Health Service would lead to less demand for medical services would not be realised. Screening tests for diseases were developed, including a range of tests on children to identify possible problems such as some metabolic diseases and hearing tests. Women were invited for breast and cervical screening.

By the 1950s smoking had become increasingly popular among both men and women. Advertising used film stars to promote cigarettes and there were even claims that cigarettes were good for your health. Public knowledge about the health risks was very poor. By the 1960s the fight against infectious diseases was progressing but the rise in the number of older people was leading to more chronic diseases and the death rates from lung cancer and heart disease were increasing. An awareness of the inequalities in health experienced by different groups in society, and the recognition of environmental hazards, directed a new way of thinking about health education. In 1967 the Health Education Council was founded to co-ordinate and plan health promotion. The publication of the Black Report in 1980 gave greater impetus to tackling the inequalities in health based on social and environmental issues.

Research tip

You can find out more about the Black Report by following the links on this website: www.ucel.ac.uk

During the 1970s and 1980s the World Health Organization (WHO) took a lead in trying to widen the debate about health and health promotion. It set international targets and aspirations. However, although influential it does not have the power or resources to implement all the actions necessary to achieve its targets.

Health for All by the Year 2000 (1977)

In 1977 the WHO launched a policy framework 'Health for All by the Year 2000' (HFA2000). It set a series of targets to enable everyone to achieve a level of health which would allow them to lead socially and economically productive lives. It has formed the basis of several initiatives over subsequent years and has been reviewed by the WHO member states regularly. These are examples of some of the original targets:

- life expectancy at birth of 70 years

- maternal mortality to be reduced by 50%

- all children to receive immunisations against diphtheria, tetanus, whooping cough, measles, polio and TB

- access to clean drinking water and the safe disposal of sewage

- access to appropriate nutrition

- primary health care to be available to all

- adult literacy rates to be at least 70%.

National governments were expected to implement the policy as most appropriate for their population. However it meant that there was an emphasis on what has been called the 'new public health'. The importance of public health measures in eliminating malnutrition, contaminated water supplies, certain diseases, and poor housing as well as providing education was recognised as different aspects of health promotion.

Alma-Ata Declaration of 1978

An international conference on primary health care was held in Alma Ata in the USSR in September 1978. The Declaration of Alma Ata stressed the importance of primary health care and this has been the major way that Health for All has been promoted. The declaration contained the following statement:

The Conference strongly reaffirms that health, which is a state of complete physical, mental and social wellbeing, and not merely the absence of disease or infirmity, is a fundamental human right and that the attainment of the highest possible level of health is a most important world-wide social goal whose realization requires the action of many other social and economic sectors in addition to the health sector.

Research tip

You can find out more about the Alma-Ata Declaration by following this link www.who.int/hpr/NPH/docs/declaration_almaata.pdf

Ottawa Charter for Health Promotion 1986

In 1986 the WHO held the first international conference on health promotion in Ottawa, Canada. This was the first of a series of conferences which outlined the international programmes of action for health promotion. The conference in Canada produced the Ottawa Charter for Health Promotion. The main areas of the declaration to promote health were:

- building a healthy public policy

- developing personal skills

- strengthening community action

- creating supportive environments

- re-orientating health care services.

Three ways in which health can be promoted were identified as

- Advocacy. Environments need to be created in which people's understanding about health is promoted so that individuals are empowered to demand the necessary changes.

- Enablement. All individuals should be enabled to achieve their full health potential. This could be through providing knowledge and skills.

- Mediation. Health promoters may need to mediate between different interested parties in order to maximise the health of a population.

MODELS

Health education is part of an overall strategy to improve health and prevent disease. We are now going to look in detail at two models of health education: that of 'victim blaming' and that of empowerment.

Key words

Victim blaming – holding the victims of an illness or accident to be in whole or in part responsible for what has happened to them

'Victim blaming' model

Initially, public health measures aimed to improve the health of individuals. Improved sanitation and housing, and the implementation of immunisation programmes, led to the reduction of many infectious diseases. As a consequence the diseases associated with the way a person chooses to live became a challenge to health professionals. The focus of health education became lifestyle choices such as alcohol consumption, smoking, physical inactivity, weight control as well as sexually transmitted diseases. This meant that the person could be held responsible for their own health rather than economic, environmental or social factors that affect health. This is known as victim blaming. In these circumstances someone with heart disease who smokes and is overweight can be blamed for the fact that they have had a heart attack. Someone who attempts suicide may be blamed for their actions. Other issues which have led to the situation, such as lack of education, poor housing, unemployment or stress, may be ignored.

Health education campaigns that take a victim blaming approach hold the individuals responsible for the health problems that they are experiencing. It may lead to health professionals ignoring or failing to react appropriately to individuals who are ill.

Example

Sean is 48 years old and now unemployed. He started work in a large manufacturing company when he left school at 16. His girlfriend, Jemma, became pregnant when they were both 17 and they got married. They now have five children and live in a three-bedroom house on a deprived estate on the edge of the city. Sean's parents both smoked and made no attempt to dissuade him when he started to smoke at 13 years old. He likes to have a drink with his mates for relaxation and as an escape from the pressures at home. Five years ago Sean lost his job when the company went into liquidation. He has found it impossible to find another job and has become more and more depressed. He spends a lot of his time now just watching the television. He and Jemma find it difficult to pay their bills as the children are often in need of clothes and shoes. They buy food as cheaply as possible. Sean has put on a lot of weight and was very frightened when he woke up one night with pains in his chest. He went to see the doctor who thinks that he may have had a heart attack. The doctor suggested that he might have brought it on himself by smoking, being overweight and not taking exercise. He said that he must take responsibility for improving his lifestyle if he wanted to get better.

> *Think* Why is this an example of victim blaming? What other factors could have caused Sean to have a heart attack?

Empowerment model

This approach aims to help people to identify their own health concerns and then work with them to develop the skills and confidence that are required. It puts the individual or client at the centre and the health educator becomes a facilitator. The clients or patients are seen as equals and have a right to set their own agenda. It is a 'bottom up' strategy with the client making the decisions about what is important. The health educator will work with the client to provide support and to give the education and training that are identified as necessary to achieve the outcomes that are wanted.

Example

Aisha is a health promotion worker employed by a Primary Care Trust. She has been asked to visit a local Sure Start group which is targeted at young mothers. She decides that she will plan a six-week programme based around good parenting, including the recommended immunisation programme and an understanding of the most common childhood diseases. When she meets the group for the first time they tell her that they would like a programme on nutrition and want to learn how to cook nourishing food for their children. Until now they have bought ready-made meals so it will mean going back to basics. Aisha is rather taken aback as it means that she will need to work with the mothers to develop a completely different programme.

> *Think* What will be the advantages and disadvantages of undertaking a health education campaign as requested by the mothers?

APPROACHES TO HEALTH EDUCATION

Health education can be undertaken in a number of different ways. The most appropriate approach will depend on the topic, the target group, the resources available and the skills of the health educator as well as other variables. We will now examine the main approaches to health education: social marketing, the role of the mass media, community development and two-way communication.

> **Key words**
>
> Social marketing – applying marketing principles in order to achieve a change in attitudes or behaviours for a social good

SOCIAL MARKETING

Marketing mix

Social marketing is applying marketing principles in order to achieve a change in attitudes or behaviours for a social good. Social marketing was first defined in the 1970s by Kotler and Zaltman who suggested that the same marketing techniques that 'sold' products to consumers could be used to 'sell' ideas, attitudes and behaviour. The concept was then applied to the idea of promoting behaviour which would positively affect health by using commercial marketing techniques. Changing the behaviour of people does not always rely on convincing them through giving factual information. Individuals do things for emotional and other reasons. Marketing uses both these approaches. It is therefore argued that the same can be applied to 'selling' the idea of health and healthy lifestyles. It moves away from simply trying to convey rational factual information and combines it with appealing to other values.

This approach relies on using what is called the marketing mix. This is a range of strategies used to sell things to people and which are known as the five 'P's:

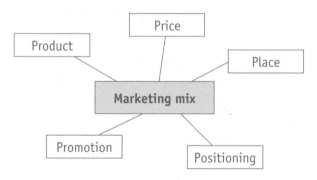

Figure 20.2 The marketing mix

The product refers to the behaviour or attitude that the audience needs to adopt. It therefore needs to be attractive, quantifiable and accessible. The price of the product includes the monetary and non-monetary cost, for example the psychological or social cost. The place means the sites where the product can be found. The more places where the product can be 'bought'

the better chance there is of the product being successfully marketed. The promotion is the way in which the awareness of the product is raised. This may be by advertising, direct marketing or other techniques. The mass media is used very frequently in social marketing and we will be exploring its role in greater depth later. Positioning relates to the image of the product and how it is linked to other issues. For example giving up smoking can be linked to better skin and a healthier complexion.

> **Key words**
> --
> Mass media – any printed or audio visual material designed to reach as mass audience

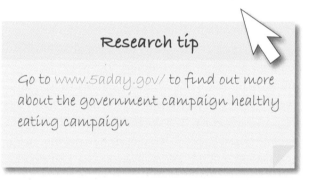

Research tip

Go to www.5aday.gov/ to find out more about the government campaign healthy eating campaign

> **Think** How could the five 'P's of the social marketing theory be applied to this '5 a Day' campaign?

Social marketing evolved as a concept because health education was previously seen as rather boring – trying to make people give up things that they enjoyed. The marketing philosophy is that the customer is always right and must be listened to. Social marketing therefore means that any health campaign must be developed with the wants and needs of the target audience kept at the centre of the plans, i.e. it will become needs-led.

Products are rarely targeted to be sold to all of the general public. Any marketing strategy will carefully analyse who should be targeted and why. Different groups are selected as the most appropriate to be persuaded to 'buy' a product and then the message is specifically targeted at them. This is known as audience segmentation. The target audience is segmented into groups that are similar to each other; for example by age or behaviour. Messages are then created which they will specifically relate to. These aspects of using the social marketing approach can be very beneficial; they help to ensure that resources are much more directed and more likely to achieve results.

Limitations

However, there are some disadvantages of following the model. The concept of a needs-led approach dictated by the customer means that sometimes these needs do not match up with the requirements shown up through academic or epidemiological research. Some 'products' may be difficult to 'market' as they are less tangible, such as 'taking more exercise'. The ability of individuals to undertake a new behaviour might be limited by their lack of skills. Marketing is also a costly activity both in resources and time. Commercial organisations can invest in high profile marketing of their goods because they expect to see a commercial return. The return from health education social marketing may be long term and at times difficult to quantify.

Example

Newtown College is a popular FE college on the edge of a large town and draws students from a wide area. It attracts people because of its relaxed atmosphere and its academic achievements. Individuals from a range of different cultural backgrounds mix together happily. The majority of the students are aged 16 to 19 years. There are more than 100 staff. There are more females than males on the campus. It has good facilities with a canteen and a sports centre.

Think Using a social marketing approach, what health needs might be targeted? How might the principles of audience segmentation be applied?

ROLE OF THE MASS MEDIA

Different forms

The mass media refers to any printed or audio-visual material designed to reach a mass audience. This includes television, radio, newspapers, magazines, posters, billboard displays, leaflets and – increasingly – the internet. Its use as a way of approaching health education has both advantages and disadvantages. It can have a wide and very powerful impact. It can convey uncomplicated information and raise the public's consciousness about health issues. Although sometimes the mass media can shock people into changing their attitudes or behaviour, evidence has shown that its effect is often short lived. For example, every Christmas there is a hard-hitting campaign against drink driving but people often ignore the message or the impact wears off over time. If it is part of an integrated campaign it can change behaviour but it cannot teach skills. There is no personal link with the mass audience, so limiting two-way communication.

The mass media can be used to promote health, for example, in the following ways.

National or regional health education campaigns

These campaigns may use the mass media, including advertisements by the major health promotion agencies using television, radio, magazines or newspapers. Advertising campaigns have addressed issues such as influenza protection, safe drinking and healthy eating.

Healthy options

'Healthy' products and services can be promoted by commercial organisations as part of the marketing strategy for their own goods. Advertisements will highlight certain properties that can be seen as 'healthy' e.g. 'low fat'. Companies such as Tesco or other supermarket chains may produce educational leaflets linked to their 'healthy eating' products. Leisure facilities may emphasise the links with exercise and health while restaurant chains advertise 'healthy' options.

Discussions/reports on health issues

Books, magazines, television and radio often have articles about health. Some magazines and books may be entirely centred on health issues while others have health among other issues of interest to their readers. Television programmes may promote health messages. Jamie Oliver, the celebrity chef, undertook a series on school meals and the findings have resulted in major changes to nutritional standards in schools.

Issues about health can also be raised indirectly as part of story lines in television or radio. This most frequently occurs in 'soaps' such as EastEnders and programmes such as Heartbeat set in a medical context. News items can reflect issues about health and contribute to people's knowledge and understanding.

Celebrities

Health experiences and behaviour by personalities who feature in the media can affect the behaviour and views of others, particularly if they are role models for certain groups. The attitudes to alcohol and drugs among sports personalities may have an effect on young people who seek to copy their lifestyle.

Sponsorship

Commercial companies have realised the advantages of being linked with health and have sought to sponsor events and people. Many sports events and personalities have sponsors, such as the English football and cricket teams. In the past, cigarette manufacturers were sponsors of sport but this has declined as it was accepted that the messages were contradictory in terms of good health.

> **Think** What do you think might be the problems for motor racing to be sponsored by a cigarette manufacturing company?

Advantages of using mass media

It:

- raises awareness about health issues
- puts health on the public agenda effecting societal change
- increases knowledge
- influences attitude and behaviour change
- has immediate emotional effect.

Disadvantages of using mass media

These can include:

- responses may be short term
- it cannot convey complex information
- it cannot teach skills
- it may only change attitudes or behaviour if in combination with other enabling factors
- some mass media stories may convey negative messages about health promotion.

COMMUNITY DEVELOPMENT

Community-based work involves the health educator working directly with a group of people to improve their health. This can be with an organisation or a community. It might be a women's group or a community living in a particular area, a cultural group or another group of people united by some shared interest or common situation.

Holistic concept

Community development starts with health needs that are identified by the community itself. This often means that health is defined quite broadly. It may include the social, economic and environmental aspects of people's lives as well as their physical or mental health. It therefore views health much more holistically. The root causes of ill health become the focus rather than the symptoms.

Participation and empowerment

In order to make improvements, community development requires participation in the process. This in itself can lead to people gaining in self confidence, improving self esteem and feeling in control. In this way people become empowered.

Community development can mean working with disadvantaged groups who experience health inequalities. This can lead to the reduction in these inequalities by tackling some of the root causes of poor health. However, the work in community development projects can be very time consuming as the health educator works with the group to build up the skills and confidence of the participants. It is also difficult to measure success.

Key words

Community development – a community defining its own needs and decides collectively how these needs should be met

CASE STUDY: PILTON COMMUNITY HEALTH PROJECT

In 1984 the Pilton Community Health Project based in the north of Edinburgh was established. It uses a community development approach to enable local people to identify their health needs and works with them to tackle the issues that affect their health, for example by campaigning or developing local resources and services. A major community consultation was undertaken and the following were identified as their objectives:

1. To alleviate the high levels of stress experienced by local people.
2. To identify, tackle and improve the life circumstances that underlie poor health.
3. To ensure local equity of access to health related services, resources and information.
4. To alleviate the high levels of isolation and loneliness experienced by older people.
5. To promote and support healthy patterns of living and healthy environments.
6. To ensure people receive support and have the opportunity to explore feelings associated with loss and bereavement.
7. To address issues relating to food poverty and healthy eating.

One of the groups set up is 'Women Supporting Women' which aims to develop a community-based service for local women who are isolated, experiencing mental distress (including depression after the birth of a baby) or who have experience of violence. This is how they describe themselves:

Women Supporting Women developed from an idea that a group of local women had in 1992. Originally focusing on postnatal depression, the project has been informed by the women who have used its services over the years and now offers a range of provision including one-to-one support, group work opportunities and a befriending service. The project also campaigns on a range of women's health issues, including postnatal depression and violence against women.

Who is it for?
Women Supporting Women primarily targets women living in Greater Pilton. If you have ever felt down, depressed or isolated, then our services might help. Many women tell us that they feel unhappy, tearful, anxious or worried, irritable or frustrated, exhausted physically and emotionally, angry or guilty, or any combination of these feelings. The feelings may arrive all at once or may develop over time. You may feel alone and that no-one understands. We offer a range of opportunities including confidence building, women's health, relationships, women's lives and much more! We provide free childcare and can pay your travel expenses.

QUESTIONS

1. Identify what health needs the community thought were important.

2. In what ways does the women's group follow the main principles of community development?

Advantages and disadvantages

Advantages may be that it:

- is user led

- tackles root causes of ill health

- leads to skills which can be transferable.

The disadvantages may be that:

- only small groups can be catered for

- it is time consuming

- the results are not always measurable.

> ### Research tip
>
> You can find out more about this project by looking at their website: www.pchp.org.uk

TWO-WAY COMMUNICATION

Communication is a two-way process involving the sending and receiving of messages. The ways in which people communicate in health and care settings and the factors that influence the effectiveness of communication are explored in detail in Unit 1. The same principles apply when undertaking health education. As a summary: communication can occur in a variety of ways including through individual and group interactions, verbal and non-verbal messages, images and graphics, technology, written communications and therapeutic activities.

There are different approaches that can be used for two-way communication. It may occur in a one-to-one situation, in small or large group settings, through the use of peer educators, using drama or role play or through interactive video and computer packages. It is part of the role of the health educator to decide what is the most effective and appropriate method to use.

One-to-one communication may be most appropriate when communicating with an individual about something that is specific to them or when giving sensitive or difficult information. Counselling may also take place on an individual basis; for example, specific health advice about a diagnosis or treatment or developing a skill or coping strategy. Health visitors visit new mothers on an individual basis to give advice about the care of their newborn baby. They will also encourage them to attend health clinics where they will receive further advice and the baby will receive appropriate immunisations.

> ### Example
>
> Jade and Lenny are planning to live together and may want to start a family. Jade's brother has a degenerative disease and she is not sure whether it is hereditary. She is going to see their G.P. to find out what she can before trying to have a baby.

> **Think** Why would it be appropriate for Jade to see her GP on a one-to one basis?

Groups can be used when giving general advice on a topic, providing information and improving knowledge. Working with groups can help to boost confidence and empower the participants. It can also be used to change attitudes and behaviour. Groups can be small or large but two-way communication can be facilitated in a number of ways to ensure that all participants are fully involved.

> ### Example
>
> Hina is a school nurse. Each year she runs health education classes on safe sex. These usually take place as part of the school's PSHE programme. She finds that they are usually very lively occasions and she likes to get the boys and girls to ask questions. She talks to them about condom use as well as the Pill and other methods of contraception. She wants them to understand about sexually transmitted diseases and the long-term consequences of unsafe sexual practices. Hina sometimes wonders if it would be better to teach the boys and girls separately.

Think What are the main objectives of Hina's lessons? In what ways could she ensure that successful two-way communication takes place?

Groups who share similar interests may also come together. This could include older people, pregnant women or groups of unemployed or those with disabilities. Communication about health matters that are specific to their needs can be given and ideas exchanged.

Think What health education messages would be most appropriate for each of the following groups or individuals?
- mothers with children under school age
- a group of women in a residential home
- a youth group for 14 to 16-year-olds
- a 50-year-old man who has just come out of hospital following a heart attack
- a Brownie pack.

In what ways could the message be given?

Peer educators

Research has shown that people are more likely to listen to health education messages if they believe that the educator is similar to them and faces the same concerns and pressures. Peer education is used to encourage healthier behaviour among young people. It is about using young people's influence over one another to make positive interventions in young people's lives. Peer education works on the principle that young people are more likely to be influenced by members of their own group of friends rather than others, particularly if they are adults or in positions of authority. Peer educators receive special training and information which they pass on to their friends. This can be particularly appropriate in supporting young people to make healthy decisions about sex.

Key words

Peer education – education to people by individuals of their own age.

CASE STUDY: ARMENIA: PEER EDUCATION, NOT FEAR EDUCATION

Armenia is considered a country with a low prevalence of HIV/AIDS but the number of those infected is growing. In 2001, surveys of young people indicated that although there was a high level of understanding regarding the importance of practising safer sex, behaviour can be just the opposite. They knew of the dangers of HIV/AIDS, but very few knew about preventive measures. Instead, most teenagers received their information from unreliable sources such as films or from friends.

Any visitor to School No. 43 in the Armenian capital might easily mistake Veronica Seropyan for a teacher standing in front of thirteen pupils aged between fourteen and sixteen. Veronica is a member of the AIDS Prevention, Education and Care (APEC) project that has charged itself with the task of training 1,400 schoolchildren as peer educators. Through interactive teaching methods, discussion and games, the children learn about the danger of infection from HIV/AIDS.

'We talk about the history of the disease,' says Veronica Seropyan, 'and how it is spread, what effect it has on the immune system as well as the biological and psychological development of teenagers. Later, they will pass on that knowledge by talking with their friends and classmates.'

QUESTIONS

1. Why do you think peer education might be successful here?

2. In what other areas might peer education work well?

Research tip

You can find out more from Emil Sahakyan, Communication Officer, UNICEF Armenia: www.unicef.org/armenia/reallives_2353.html

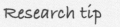

Research tip

Log on to NHS Direct to get health information at www.nhsdirect.nhs.uk

Theatre and drama

Another way of approaching health education is through the use of theatre and drama. Messages can be conveyed directly or indirectly as part of a story line. The development of skills and confidence can often be enhanced through the use of drama. Sensitive subjects may be expressed through drama; for example, theatre groups have spread health messages among Mozambique's flood victims.

Finally as computers and videos become more interactive they can be used as a method of two-way communication. Interactive packages offer health assessments. Video can facilitate live discussions and may be used to provide information.

EVIDENCE ACTIVITY

P1 – M1

P1 Explain three different approaches to health education.

M1 Compare three different approaches to health education.

Choose three health education campaigns that use different approaches. Describe and compare each of the campaigns, including the subject matter and the approach that is used. Were they appropriate for the campaign and why was one approach chosen above another?

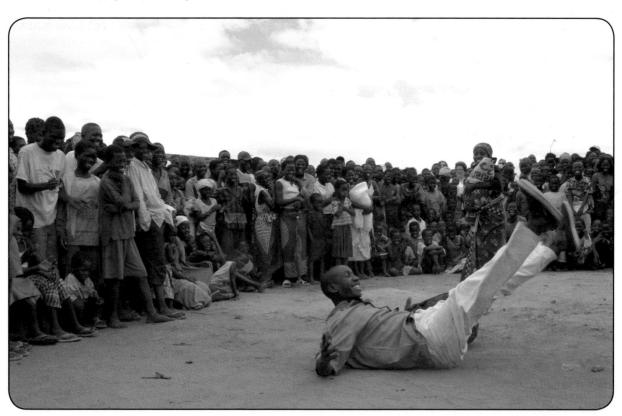

Figure 20.3 Children in Mozambique, captivated by a play, learn important skills from community activists.

20.2 *Understand models of behaviour change*

MODELS

The ultimate aim of any health education is to change people's behaviour so that they lead healthier lives. However, it is not always straightforward to get individuals to adopt healthy behaviours and the process of making any change can be complex. The various stages through which individuals change are described in a number of different models.

Health belief model

The health belief model is one of the best known. It suggests that:

- an individual must believe that they are susceptible to a certain disease

- the disease is serious

- the proposed preventative action will be beneficial

- the benefits will outweigh any costs or disadvantages

- they are competent to carry out the behaviour

- the likelihood of action will be enhanced if the individual has a positive view of health

- cues or triggers to action are provided.

Example

Simon is in his first year at university. He is shocked to hear that one of his fellow students has developed meningitis and is very ill. The university has distributed a number of leaflets giving information about the disease. Simon realises that his age group is at particular risk. The medical centre is offering immunisation to all students. However Simon does not like needles.

Think Use the health belief model to see if you can predict whether Simon will attend the medical centre and why.

Theory of reasoned action

Fishbein and Ajzen proposed the theory of reasoned action. They suggested that behaviour can be predicted by knowing what someone intends to do. An intention is formed by a person's attitude to the behaviour and their perception of what other people will think about them if they behave in a certain way (subjective norms). This model recognises that the attitudes of other people can also have an effect on the behaviour of an individual.

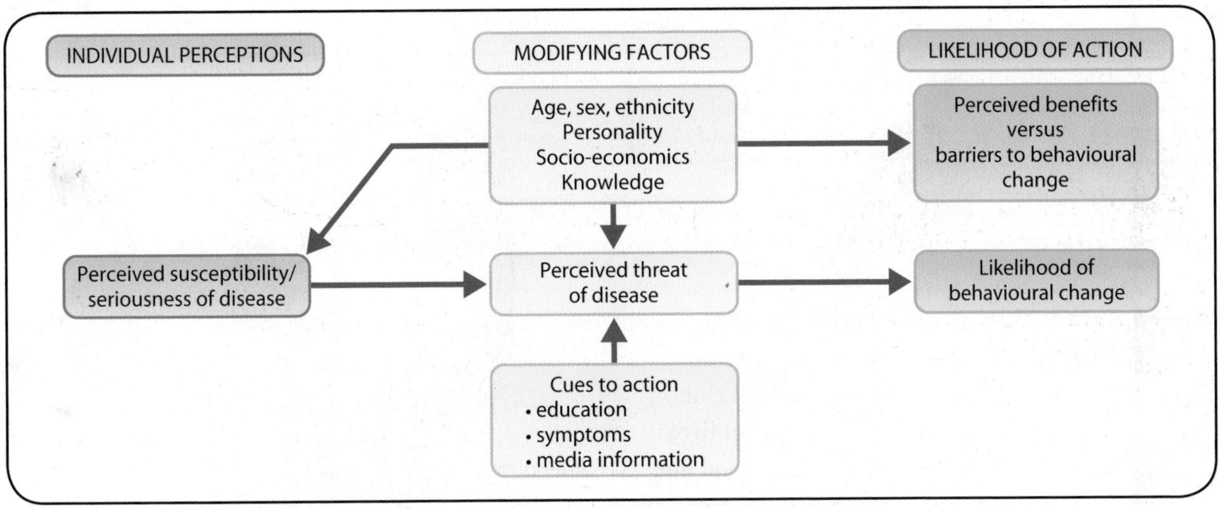

Figure 20.4 The health belief model (Source: Glanz, K., Rimer, B.K. & Lewis, F.M. (2002). Health Behavior and Health Education. Theory, Research and Practice. San Fransisco: Wiley & Sons)

Example

Sonya has moved to a new area and is keen to make new friends. She has never smoked and neither do her parents. She is keen on sports and wants to stay fit. Her brother has the occasional cigarette and she has helped him to avoid being caught by their parents. After her first week at school she is invited out to a friend's house on Saturday night. When she arrives she finds all her new friends are smoking and they assume that she will join in with them.

Think Using the theory of reasoned action, consider whether or not Sonya is likely to smoke.

Theory of planned behaviour

Ajzen built on the theory of reasoned action to develop his theory of planned behaviour, which added a third influence – behavioural control. This reflects an individual's perceptions of their ability to perform certain behaviour. So behaviour is governed by behavioural intentions, which are influenced by the individual's attitude and how they think other people view the behaviour, and also the individual's beliefs about how easy it will be for them to undertake the behaviour, for example whether they have the skills or resources to act in a certain way.

Research tip

To find out more about this theory go to www.people.umass.edn/aizen/

Example

Paul wants to improve his fitness. He has been trying to decide what activity he should take up. Some of his mates belong to a local football club and have been encouraging him to join. Paul likes football but is not sure whether he is any good and does not want to make a fool of himself. In addition to this, the training ground is some distance away and he is not sure if he can get a lift.

Think Using the theory of planned behaviour, do you think Paul is likely to take up football to improve his fitness?

Stages of change model

The stages of change model was developed by Prochaska and DiClemente, who had been working with smokers trying to give up their addiction. They suggested that in order to change behaviour individuals went through various stages. These were identified as:

- Precontemplation. At this stage the individual has a problem which they may or may not recognize. However they have not considered changing their behaviour and are not aware of any risks associated with the behaviour.

- Contemplation. The individual is aware of the problem and of the benefits of changing their behaviour. They may be seeking information to help make a decision about changing.

- Preparation to change. The problem is recognised and the individual is ready to change. They may seek extra support to help them make the change

- Making the change. The individual changes their behaviour. They may have a clear goal and plans including support and rewards.

- Maintenance. The new behaviour is sustained.

- Relapse may occur in which case the individual may rejoin the cycle.

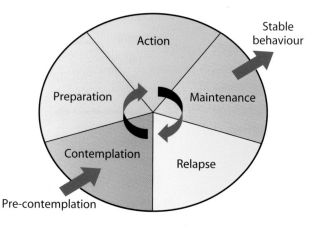

Figure 20.5 Stages of change model, Prochaskae Di and Clemente

Example

Alan is a businessman. As part of his job he regularly meets clients over a drink in the evening and he has clinched some important deals at these times. Alan has never been concerned about the amount of alcohol that he drinks. He sees it as a normal part of his life. His partner reckons that he probably has the equivalent of a bottle of wine each night and more at the weekend. Apply the theory of stages of change to changing Alan's behaviour towards alcohol.

Social learning theory

The social learning theory was developed by the psychologist Bandura. He suggested that behaviour can be explained by the way in which three factors continually interact: the environmental, personal and behavioural factors. People learn to behave in certain ways not only through their own experiences but also by observing others and the consequences of their actions. Human behaviour is learned through watching others and modelling the behaviour of others particularly those who are regarded as role models. This is frequently used in television commercials where a product is associated with an outcome that is valued; for example, the drinking of a certain beverage is linked with social acceptance. This may well result in the behaviour of drinking the product being modelled.

Example

The Italian fashion capital has formally barred ultra-skinny and under-age models ahead of its February catwalk shows, as the fashion world comes under pressure to promote a healthier image. In December 2006 an agreement was signed between the city and its powerful fashion industry to ban from the shows models under 16 and those with a body mass index of less than 18.5.

Think Can you apply the principles of social learning theory to the story about skinny models?

IMPORTANCE OF SOCIAL AND ECONOMIC CONTEXT

Health education does not take place in a vacuum but within the context of social and economic settings. All programmes for health-related behaviour change have a cost in terms of resources – money, time or social and emotional factors. Sometimes results are difficult to measure and so the cost effectiveness cannot be clearly measured. In financial terms, a cost benefit analysis may be undertaken before embarking on a programme. For example, the cost of the breast screening programme in the UK runs into many millions of pounds. However the early detection of cancer has saved many women's lives and prolonged the lives of others. Other interventions may have much longer term results. Stopping a young person from smoking will affect the chances of avoiding heart and lung disease much later in life. But putting a price on health outcomes is very difficult.

Think National No Smoking Day aims to help people to stop smoking. How can it be assessed whether the methods are cost effective in helping smokers to stop?

Financial and social constraints

Finances for health care are always under great demand. Health education programmes have to compete for money in the NHS and from other health and social care providers. Advertising and the use of the mass media is very costly and unlike commercial organisations the return on investments are not easily quantifiable.

For the individual there may be financial implications to changing their behaviour. Health-related activities such as swimming or going to the gym may involve the cost of membership or entrance fees. Changes in diet to more healthy options may require more money.

Social factors may also prove a constraint. The influence of others may be the deciding factor that either supports or discourages a change in behaviour. Some changes may mean a change in lifestyle, including social activities.

Example

Cathy has three children. She is unemployed and lives on benefits. She sometimes finds it difficult to make ends meet. But she has some good friends and they all meet up regularly to have a chat and a smoke and so the children can play together. Last winter her youngest child had a chest infection and was hospitalised. She was very poorly for a few days. The hospital said that her resistance was low and she needed to have a healthy nourishing diet and be kept away from smoky atmospheres. Cathy was very shocked by her daughter's illness and wants to do all she can to avoid it happening again.

Think What financial and social constraints are there on changing Cathy's behaviour?

Peer pressure

Peer pressure is the influence of a social group on an individual to conform to the behaviours of the group. Children and teenagers are the most vulnerable to peer pressure. It can influence how they dress, the music they listen to and the behaviours they adopt. This includes health behaviour and risk-taking activities such as drug taking, smoking, drinking and sexual activity.

EVIDENCE ACTIVITY

P2

Read through the different models of behaviour change and for each model identify a health education campaign that has used the model. Suggest what social and economic factors may have influenced the planning and implementation of each campaign.

For P2 you need to make sure that you have described two different models of behaviour change and the importance of the social and economic context.

20.3 Know how health education campaigns are implemented.

This section explores the principles of implementing a health education campaign and you will also be encouraged to apply the principles to your own health activity. This forms part of the assessment of this unit. It should be fun to plan and carry out – so start thinking of a health topic that interests you.

HEALTH EDUCATORS

Health education is not limited to one organisation but crosses the boundaries between education, the environment and social issues as well as the health services. Therefore people who are involved in educating for health may come from any of these sectors. A doctor or health visitor may give health advice as part of their professional work but so may a teacher in school or an environmental health officer. Sometimes different organisations may work together forming 'healthy alliances'. This accords with the views expressed by the WHO in its document 'Health For All by the year 2000'.

Health for all requires the coordinated action of all sectors concerned. The health authorities can only deal with a part of the problems to be solved and multisectoral cooperation is the only way of effectively ensuring the perquisites for health, promoting health policies and reducing the risks in the physical, economic and social environment.' (WHO 1985)

International

As well as the World Health Organization, other international organisations are involved in health education. The WHO has a role that is specifically aimed at monitoring and improving the health of all countries. It has been instrumental in shifting the emphasis from a medical base to primary health care. This has meant promoting health in its broadest definition and directing action at ensuring the environment supports healthy living. The United Nations and the European Union have all issued directives which concern the health of their member countries. These include setting standards or targets and developing initiatives on issues which include cancer prevention, pollution, HIV/AIDS, diet and social inequalities.

Research tip

UNICEF is one of many international organisations dedicated to improving health. Go to their website to find out more www.unicef.org

National

In the national context the Department of Health naturally takes the lead on health. Within the Department of Health the NHS (National Health Service) is the major agency for promoting health. However, the Department of Health needs to work with other government departments such as that for Education and Science, Transport, the Environment and the Home Office which also contribute to health promotion in a variety of ways. The lead agency in health promotion – the Health Development Agency – has combined with the Health Protection Agency under the banner of National Institute for Health and Clinical Excellence (NICE) with the remit to provide national guidance on the promotion of good health and the prevention and treatment of ill health. You can find out more about the work of the Health Protection Agency in Unit 12 page 78. Campaigns that promote health may come from different government departments. For example, drink driving campaigns are the responsibility of the Department for Transport; school meals are the responsibility of the Department of Education and healthy eating that of the NHS.

> **Think** Who might educate children about road safety?

Research tip

Go to the website to find out more about the children's road safety campaign – www.hedgehogs.gov.uk

Primary Care Trusts

Primary Care Trusts (PCTs) cover all parts of England and receive their budgets directly from the Department of Health. However, if you live in Scotland or Northern Ireland primary healthcare services are organised differently from England and Wales.

PCTs are responsible for ensuring that there are sufficient healthcare services for their local population. This includes GPs, social workers, health visitors, district nurses, school nurses, dentists, opticians and community pharmacists. They may also provide a range of community services such as services for children, adults and older people and people with disabilities; sexual and reproductive health services, foot health services, mental health services, services for carers and many more. They purchase the services which local people need from a wide range of organisations including hospitals, specialist providers of mental health services, voluntary sector and community groups as well as, increasingly, the independent sector.

The services provided in primary care are being expanded and different professionals are joining the team. It is not unusual to have counsellors and therapists attached to practices and for specialist services to be offered. All members of the primary care team have a role in health promotion. The practice nurse may run 'wellness' clinics which promote healthy living as well as screening people with chronic conditions such as diabetes. The health visitor works both with groups and on a one-to-one basis but also with a network of other professionals in education and social services. The midwife provides information and support to pregnant women and mothers and their new babies. GPs provide medical services promoting health and have the responsibility for ensuring that the practice is meeting government targets for immunisation, screening and checks for older people. There are many opportunities for health promotion that are available to them throughout the course of their work through planned interventions and opportunistically in giving advice. Pharmacists can offer further information to the client collecting a prescription and may be asked for advice about appropriate medication or treatment.

Local authorities have responsibility for planning, housing, recreation and leisure. They employ a wide range of people who will as part of their job educate people about their health. For example, youth workers can work in services which target young people who have been affected by alcohol misuse or provide leisure activities which promote health. Education authorities work with teachers and lecturers in schools and colleges in providing health education. Social workers, the police and fire service all work with their local community on health issues. For example, primary schools will often have a visit from their local community police officer to talk to the children on topics of health and safety.

Research tip

Find out about your own PCT or primary healthcare service to find out what local services you have. You could start with the Department of Health website: www.dh.gov.uk

HEALTH STRATEGIES

Information about the health of a population is collected internationally, nationally and locally. (This is covered in greater detail in Unit 12.) It is important that the health needs of populations are understood in order to set strategies to meet those needs. Within any strategy there are targets to be met and this gives the opportunity for an assessment to be made about the success or otherwise of the strategy. In 1992 the *Health of the Nation* strategy was published with five key target areas of coronary heart disease, accidents, mental health, sexual health and cancers. It was followed in 1999 by *Saving Lives – Our Healthier Nation*. In this the UK government set key targets to be achieved by the year 2010:

- cancer – to reduce the death rate in people under 75 by at least a fifth

- coronary heart disease and stroke – to reduce the death rate in people under 75 by at least two-fifths

- accidents – to reduce the death rate by at least a fifth and serious injury by at least a tenth

- mental illness – to reduce the death rate from suicide and undetermined injury by at least a fifth.

The strategy by which these targets were to be achieved included:

- putting in more money: £21 billion for the NHS alone to help secure a healthier population

- tackling smoking as the single biggest preventable cause of poor health

- integrating national and local government to work to improve health

- stressing health improvement as a key role for the NHS

- pressing for high health standards for all.

The NHS was to be 'reorientated' so that health improvement would be integrated into the local delivery of health care. This was to be achieved by:

- health authorities having a new role in improving the health of local people

- primary care groups and primary care trusts having new responsibilities for public health

- local authorities working in partnership with the NHS to plan for health improvement

- standards being measured by a new Health Development Agency, a statutory body charged with raising the standards and quality of public health provision.

There would be an increase in education and training for health, with a new skills audit and workforce development plan, and specific measures for nurses, midwives, health visitors, school nurses and others. Public health information would be improved by establishing public health observatories in each NHS region, setting up disease registers, and promoting research.

Research tip

Find out more about Saving Lives Our Healthier Nation (1999) by going to www.archive.official-documents.co.uk/document/cm43/4386/4386-sm.htm

Strategies to meet other targets for health have been developed including ones directed at alcohol harm reduction and sexually transmitted infections and the rates of unintended pregnancies.

Choosing Health

In 2004 the government launched Choosing Health – Making Healthy Choices Easier. The aim was to make it easier for people to choose to live healthy lives. The areas of smoking, obesity, exercise, alcohol consumption and sexual and mental health were identified as being the most important targets.

Poorer communities were to be particularly targeted. Sales of cigarettes, unhealthy foods and alcohol were to be restricted, especially to children and young people. Schools were encouraged to provide healthier foods, promote exercise and use school nurses to promote health. Workplaces were encouraged to help their employees to stay healthy.

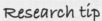

Research tip

You can view the booklet on the Department of Health website www.dh.gov.uk

Strategies targeted to different countries or localities

Information about the health status of a population may show significant differences between countries or localities even within the UK. For example the death rates from lung cancer between England and Scotland show variation. This will lead to different strategies for health education in different localities.

Look at the table below showing the number of deaths and mortality rates for lung cancer in the UK for 2005.

Table 20.1

	England	Wales	Scotland	N.Ireland	UK
Deaths					
Males	15,692	1,065	2,195	505	19,457
Females	11,119	756	1,814	319	14,008
Persons	26,811	1,821	4,009	824	33,465
Crude rate per 100,000 population					
Males	63.6	73.8	89.9	60.1	66.2
Females	43.4	49.5	69.0	36.4	45.7
Persons	53.3	61.3	79.1	48.0	55.8
Age-standardised rate (European) per 100,000 population					
Males	50.8	53.6	72.1	57.2	52.9
Females	28.7	32.0	44.6	27.8	30.2
Persons	38.3	41.1	56.2	40.4	40.0

(Source: http://info.cancerresearchuk.org)

> **Think** What does 'age-standardised rate' mean? Compare the different death rates for different parts of the UK. How could this information be used when planning health education strategies?

The role of legislation

The population is educated about health in a variety of ways. However, sometimes laws are also passed to protect individuals and ensure that their health is safeguarded. This legislation includes a wide range of health and safety regulations but also some laws which are specifically directed at individuals and their behaviours which may affect their health. There is sometimes an argument as to how far such rules might infringe an individual's right to make their own choices. However, evidence has shown that such laws can make a very big impact on health and enforce a change in society; for example the imposition of laws regarding the wearing of seat belts, helmets when riding motor cycles and, in 2007, the banning of smoking in public places.

CASE STUDY: ALEX

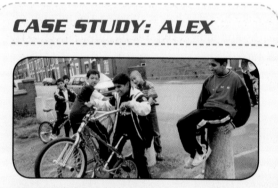

Figure 20.6 Alex and friends

Alex is a lively 12-year-old boy who likes to go out with his friends on his bike. When he was younger his parents always insisted that he wore a safety helmet. However his Dad never wore one. His school has organised cycling awareness classes which he has undertaken. The instructor encouraged them all to continue to wear their helmets. However, Alex and his friends do not think that it is 'cool' to wear a helmet when they are out together and tease one of their group who always uses his.

QUESTIONS

1. How would legislation that enforced the wearing of cycle helmets make a difference?

2. Why is it not compulsory? Do you think that it should be?

Aspects of health

In Unit 7 we explored the different aspects of health.

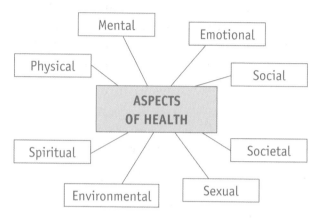

Figure 20.7 Different aspects of health

- Physical health concerns the functioning of the body

- Mental health involves the ability to think clearly and make judgements

- Emotional health relates to feelings and the ability to recognise and express them appropriately

- Spiritual health is concerned with an individual's beliefs and values, which may include religious beliefs and how they put them into practice.

- Social health is the satisfactory interaction with other people

- Sexual health is the acceptance and expression of individual sexuality

- Societal health is a wider aspect which affects the individual. The way individuals are treated within a society will affect health whether it is because of the lack of basic necessities or through racism, political unrest, war or inequalities between men and women

- Environmental health is the standard of physical environment in which individuals live including housing, sanitation and pollution.

Health education campaigns may be targeted at one or two aspects or seek to address health holistically by including all aspects of health.

AIMS AND OBJECTIVES

Before starting any health education programme it is important to determine the main aims and objectives and what methods are the most appropriate to use. The overall aim will be to improve the health of individuals and society. But this can be done in different ways such as:

- providing health-related learning

- exploring values and attitudes

- providing knowledge and skills for change

- promoting self esteem and empowerment

- changing beliefs, attitudes, behaviour or lifestyle.

Learning has three main aspects: cognitive, which is about knowledge and understanding; affective, which is concerned with attitudes and feelings; and behavioural which covers skills. In order to help people learn about health we need to cover the three aspects of learning.

Health-related learning seeks to provide information about health. This will require good communication skills and a range of methods can be used. For example talks, displays and exhibitions, written materials and the mass media are all ways of conveying information and so teaching people about their health.

Values and attitudes to health can be explored by seeking to understand how people feel about their health and the values that they put on it. This can be done through such activities as discussions or one-to-one counselling that allows individuals to express their views which can then be taken into consideration when planning a health education campaign.

As well as providing information about health, in order for people to make changes they need to have the skills to make that change. They can then make an informed choice. Decision-making skills

can be developed through activities or role play where people can practise the skills they may need. For example, in the 1990s there was a campaign to discourage children from taking drugs called 'Just Say No' which offered suggestions for various ways in which they could refuse to take drugs.

Empowerment helps people to be able to identify and express their own concerns and have the skills to act upon them. In order to meet the aim of self empowerment the health educator needs to work with clients to develop skills which increase their self esteem and therefore enable them to have greater control over their lives. This can be achieved through working in groups, treating clients as equals and facilitating any actions that the group identifies.

The ultimate aim of changing beliefs, attitudes, behaviour and lifestyles may need to involve a range of different strategies which build on each other. You can look back to page 162 to see the different models of health education and what each model aims to do.

CONTEXT

Health education can be delivered in different contexts. The mass media seeks to target large groups of people. This may be because the message is suited to large sections of the population. Other campaigns may be directed at different groups. These groups will have been identified through analysis of epidemiological data or other sources. They will have particular characteristics which may need to be taken into account when planning the campaign, for example different cultural or ethnic backgrounds, different age, sex or socio-economic status. Materials may be more appropriate for some groups rather than others. In certain circumstances one-to-one meetings may be the most appropriate way of ensuring that an individual receives the health education message appropriately.

Aim	Appropriate method
Health awareness goal	Talks Group work Mass media Displays and exhibitions Campaigns
Improving knowledge Providing information	1-to-1 teaching Displays and exhibitions Written material Mass media Campaigns Group teaching
Self empowering Improving self awareness, self esteem, decision making	Group work Practising decision making Values clarification Social skills training Simulation and role play Assertiveness training Counselling
Changing attitudes and behaviours Changing the lifestyles of individuals	Group work Skills training Self help groups 1-to-1 instruction Group or individual therapy Written material Advice

Table 20.2 Aims and methods in health promotion [Adapted from Aims and methods in health promotion Promoting health a practical guide Ewles and Simnett. Scutari Press 1985]

DESIGN PRINCIPLES

When you are designing any health education campaign, whether large or small, certain principles have to be followed. Your small-scale activity should therefore follow the same steps as one that is a large or government-funded campaign. The resources and audience may be very different but the principles are much the same. You need to follow these points carefully in order to be successful! A detailed plan will help to structure the different stages and provide a framework to keep the programme to time and linked with the original aim.

Importance of a health policy

First it is important to identify a particular aspect of health and the health education policy with which it is associated. There are many aspects of health that can benefit from a health education campaign. The government and other agencies have policies which indicate the main standards for particular aspects of health and they may publish policy guidelines. For example you might wish to consider exercise; so you will need to understand the policy regarding the right amount of exercise for health. What are the recommended guidelines for exercise for different age groups?

Gathering information

When you have decided on an aspect of health and considered the associated policy, the planning will move on to identifying the needs and priorities in that area. Any decision to undertake a health education campaign must be supported through evidence, including finding and analysing facts and statistics; for example, the causes and effects of a condition. Any information about the likelihood of individuals getting a disease, the statistics relating to illness and death from certain conditions, and the attitudes of individuals to healthy behaviours may all be relevant. This can be done through secondary research – finding and analysing reports of research carried out by others, which may include epidemiological data. Alternatively, it may be through undertaking primary research when the health educator finds out new research for themselves.

Target setting

The overall aim of the campaign will influence its planning and delivery. Specific objectives will identify how the aim is to be achieved. These should be **smart**:

- **s**pecific – clearly defined
- **m**easurable – able to be quantified
- **a**chievable – can be completed
- **r**ealistic – appropriate for the circumstances
- **t**imebound – have timings for completion.

It is particularly important when undertaking a small-scale activity to understand the constraints of working in this way and to set appropriate objectives. For example, it would not be appropriate to aim to change the behaviour of all the girls in a school if the promotion is only directed at one year group. Information must be targeted at the right age group in the most effective way. For example, handing out detailed leaflets on dental hygiene would not be the most effective way of teaching young children how to clean their teeth!

Choice of approach

Once the aim and objectives have been set, it is necessary to choose the best approach to meet them. Look back at the table on page 180 (Aims and methods in health promotion) which will give some guidance as to what methods are most appropriate for which aim. The decision may also be influenced by considering which approach would be most effective in achieving the aims of the campaign and which is most appropriate for the chosen target group, which is the easiest to use in a given situation and which is most cost effective.

Giving information

Health information can be conveyed in many different ways. Posters and leaflets are a traditional method but new technology is increasingly being used, for example text messages. As well as the medium, the tone and style can also vary. This may be particularly useful when conveying messages that may be regarded as rather personal or 'embarrassing'. In these situations a light-hearted or jokey approach might be used.

Example

Everyman is an organisation which seeks to raise awareness about male cancers such as prostate or testicular cancer. In 2006 it launched a campaign called 'Notice your Nuts' which encouraged men to check their testicles regularly for signs of testicular cancer.

Research tip

For more information on the Everyman organisation look at the website:
www.icr.ac.uk/everyman

CASE STUDY: JENNA

Jenna is a health visitor. Her project aims to improve the diets of young children (specifically the under-fives) in her area. This is part of the strategy of the PCT working with the local SureStart supporting young mothers. Jenna works with her nutritionist colleague to set up a programme of healthy eating for young children. She researches the subject, ensuring that she knows the guidelines and has looked at the reports from other similar projects. This has helped her to identify the resources she might need and the most appropriate group to target.

Jenna then sets one of her objectives: 'Within six weeks, to have raised the awareness of healthy eating with young mothers and have a minimum of four families following healthy diets for at least two months.'

QUESTIONS

1. How has Jenna gone about developing her health education campaign?

2. In what ways is her objective SMART?

Misinformation

Health is such an important aspect of all our lives that it is important that health information is correct and not misinterpreted. Research discoveries mean there may be changes in advice. For example, the programme for immunisation of young children has changed in the light of new research. It is important that facts are checked to ensure that they are accurate and up to date. When health educators talk to people there may be times when certain beliefs and prejudices have to be challenged. Sources of information must be checked to ensure that they are reliable and unbiased and that the information is accurate.

Inter-agency working

A health campaign may be strengthened if there is evidence of several partners working together to promote the same message. Professional groups may support each other and work together to promote health. As we have seen already, health may be influenced by social and environmental issues as well as physical and mental problems. It is therefore often essential that different agencies should work together to meet the needs of an individual or those of a community.

National campaigns

There are some national campaigns which are run every year; for example, there is a campaign before Christmas to try to reduce the number of deaths and accidents associated with drunken driving. National No Smoking Day every March sees individuals and organisations working together to spread the message and support individuals who want to give up smoking. Opportunities are sometimes taken to commit a certain month of the year to one particular aspect of health. For example, October has been designated breast cancer awareness month and many companies and organisations come together to promote the wearing of a pink ribbon and to raise money for research into breast cancer.

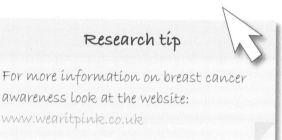

Figure 20.8 October is the month for breast cancer awareness

Research tip

For more information on breast cancer awareness look at the website: www.wearitpink.co.uk

ETHICAL CONSIDERATIONS

Health education sets out to influence people. However, not everybody has the same values and priorities. It is therefore important that certain principles should be maintained in order to ensure that any campaign is ethical. These principles follow the care value base and include:

- promoting anti-discriminatory practice
- maintaining confidentiality
- supporting the rights of individuals
- acknowledging the personal beliefs of others.

Key words

Ethics – the beliefs about what is good and bad and the code of conduct on which moral decisions are based.

Ethical considerations are necessary before starting any campaign and there may be times when difficult decisions have to be made. For example, there may be a situation about whether individual choice should take priority over the health of the whole community. Immunisation is only effective if a high level of immunity is achieved in the whole population. This means that everybody needs to participate to ensure that the whole population is safe from certain diseases.

The health educator may be in a powerful position to tailor the information to influence individuals to act in a certain way. Commercial organisations may offer to sponsor an activity in order to promote their own brand or to be associated with a good image; but this may mean that ethical questions have to be asked.

Confidentiality is always of paramount importance, particularly when questioning individuals about their own health. Messages should be checked to ensure that they promote equality of opportunity and do not stereotype or unfairly discriminate.

We will consider the rights of the individual versus the rights of others in the following case study.

Checklist

Here are some questions to consider when planning a health education campaign.

- What is the most appropriate resource for conveying my health education message?

- Who is it directed to?

- Should it be paper-based so people can read it, or take it away with them?

- What size of print and colours should be used?

- What is the best style or format?

- Would visual images enhance the message? What about photographs and video?

- Would an interactive activity be more challenging? Think about what is affordable or possible.

- What are the characteristics of the people with whom I am working?

- Is the material relevant for the people to whom it is directed? Consider their age range, gender and ethnic group. What socio-economic backgrounds do they have?

CASE STUDY: JOE'S SMOKING

Joe is 65 years old and he has smoked since he was 12. He feels he has the right to smoke at any time and in any place that he chooses. He argues that he is only hurting himself and it is his affair if he has health problems associated with smoking. His daughter, Kelly, who is a nurse, does not smoke and she is concerned about her mother who has angina. There is also her 5-year-old daughter, Amy, who likes to spend time with her grandfather. Kelly knows that children who grow up with smoking parents have more chronic respiratory diseases, such as colds, bronchitis and pneumonia, than children who grow up in non-smoking households. Patients with angina pectoris who are exposed to carbon monoxide from cigarette smoke can tolerate less exercise before experiencing chest pain. Studies now indicate that secondhand smoke may be a leading cause of lung cancer occurring in non-smokers.

QUESTIONS

1. Should Joe be allowed to continue to smoke wherever he wants?

2. What should his daughter do to try to protect his rights and the rights of others?

- Does it promote equality and diversity?

- You must ensure that there is no stereotyping or unfair discrimination. Does your message promote equality of opportunity and celebrate diversity?

- Does it contain correct information?

Check that the information is up to date and accurate. New findings may alter advice over time.

- Is it unbiased?

- Is it understandable?

- Is the information easy to understand? Is the language clear? Should it be in any other languages? Are any statistics easily understood?

- What tone – is it appropriate to use fear tactics or a light-hearted presentation?

- Will it achieve my aim?

EVALUATION

Evaluation is necessary to find out whether or not a health education campaign has been successful. This involves assessing the results and checking if the aims and objectives have been met. It is important to plan the evaluation method that will be used before starting the campaign. In order to measure any progress it may be necessary to undertake a baseline assessment to see what people know before the campaign.

The evaluation will measure not only the outcomes but also how successful – or otherwise – the methods used have been. The evidence from an evaluation should justify the use of resources and the methods used, identify any unwanted outcomes, discuss how improvements could be made and show how effective the activity has been.

The World Health Organization defined it in this way:

Evaluation implies judgment based on careful assessment and critical appraisal of given situations which should lead to drawing sensible conclusions and making useful proposals for future action.

Methods of evaluation

These can include:

- before and after questioning – this could be through questionnaires, interviews, tests or discussions

- observation of changes in behaviours or attitudes

- record of physical changes for example weight or fitness

- any changes in policy.

A self evaluation of how the individual has performed when carrying out the activity will also provide information on its success or otherwise.

	Evidence of evaluation
Aims and objectives	
Ethical issues	
Targets and strategies	
Strengths	
Weaknesses	
Potential for improvement	

A checklist for evaluation

EVIDENCE ACTIVITY

P3 – P4 – P5 – M2 – M3 – M4 – D1 – D2

The assessment activities to cover P3, P4, P5, M2, M3, M4, D1 and D2 all relate to the health education campaign that you will undertake. You may do the activity individually or as part of a small or large group. However, you must present your evidence individually.

This is your chance to put into practice many of the things that you have learned. Make sure you choose a topic that you are really interested in and start making your plan as early as possible. Choose your topic and your target group. Gather information. Plan your health education campaign including how you will evaluate it. Deliver your campaign to your chosen group. Make sure you keep good records of all you do.

For P3: Describe how you designed and implemented your health education campaign.

For M2: explain the approaches and methods that you used and relate them to the theoretical models of behaviour change.

For D1: evaluate the approaches and methods used, again making sure you relate them to the theoretical models.

For P4: explain how you met your aims and objectives and any ethical problems that were involved.

For M3: analyse how you met your aims and objectives and addressed any ethical issues.

For P5: explain how your activity links to local/national/international targets and strategies for health.

For M4: analyse the role of your activity in terms of local/national/international targets and strategies for health.

For D2: evaluate your own health education activity.

INDEX

Edexcel
190 High Holborn
London WC1V 7BH

ISBN: 978-1-40586-81-2

Printed in the Great Britain by Scotprint Ltd, Haddington
Illustrations by Pearson Education
Indexed by Richard Howard

Acknowledgments
The Publisher is grateful to the following for their permission to reproduce copyright material:

National domestic violence charity Women's Aid Federation of England; Dahlgren G, Whitehead M. 1991. Policies and Strategies to Promote Social Equity in Health" Stockholm, Sweden: Institute for Futures Studies; www.statistics.gov.uk; No Smoking Day poster, Image by Permission of No Smoking Day; Stop Look Listen Live logo reproduced with the permission of Department for Transport; Wear it Pink logo reproduced with the permission of Breast Cancer Campaign;

© Crown copyright material is reproduced with the permission of the Controller of HMSO and Queen's Printer for Scotland.

Every effort has been made to trace the copyright holders and we apologise in advance for any unintentional omissions. We would be pleased to insert the appropriate acknowledgement in any subsequent edition of this publication.

The publisher would like to thank the following for their kind permission to reproduce their photographs:

(Key: b-bottom; c-centre; l-left; r-right; t-top)

Alamy Images: Paul Doyle 137; Andrew Fox 106; Photofusion 103; **Corbis:** Beathan 10-11, 12; Burstein Collection 160; Laura Dwight 115; George Shelley 40-41, 42; John Wilkes Studio 156-157, 158; Krista Kennell/ZUMA 128-129, 130; M. Neugebauer/zefa 5t, 70-71, 72; Gideon Mendel 28; Gabe Palmer 104; Bahar Yurukoglu/Zefa 20; **Getty Images:** Photolibrary 30; Graeme Robertson 45; Taxi/Ray Kachatorian 52; **Photofusion Picture Library:** Chapman Wiedelphoto 132; Jacky Chapman 134; Paul Doyle 143; Melanie Friend 127; Judy Harrison 148; Crispin Hughes 39, 46, 108, 138; Roderick Smith 99; Sam Tanner 27; Ulrike Preuss 110, 154; Lisa Woollett 178; **Rex Features:** 122; Alix/Phanie 58; Image Source 43; **Science Photo Library Ltd:** Lauren Shear 4, 100-101, 102; **UN Photolibrary:** 26; **UNICEF/Thierry Delvigne-Jean:** UNICEF/Thierry Delvigne-Jean 5b, 170

Cover photo © Randy Faris / Corbis

All other images © Pearson Education

Picture Research by: Louise Edgeworth

Every effort has been made to trace the copyright holders and we apologise in advance for any unintentional omissions. We would be pleased to insert the appropriate acknowledgement in any subsequent edition of this publication.